As an addiction physician, I understand that recovery involves more than just quitting the drug; it also requires a spiritual component. *Life Unbinged: Faith-Filled Freedom from Food Obsession* by Kristy McCammon presents a Christian approach to tackling food addiction. McCammon, herself a food addict in recovery, shares how her faith reshaped her relationship with food. Her book provides a structured plan for treating food addiction, with practical tools and menus focusing on five essential boundaries: reliance on God, three meals daily, portion control, and eliminating sugar and flour. I am happy to endorse this book for Christians aiming for lasting recovery from food addiction.

VERA TARMAN, MD
Author of *Food Junkies: Recovery from Food Addiction*

In *Life Unbinged*, Kristy points out that surrendering to God isn't just something we do once. It must become a lifestyle. We must understand the grave importance of surrender in order to lose weight and keep it off. This book is crammed full of great resources to help you on your food addiction recovery journey. Don't miss this great book. You'll want to refer to it often.

TERESA SHIELDS PARKER
Author, coach, and podcaster

Life Unbinged is more than just a food plan—it's a path to lasting freedom from unhealthy habits. With practical tools and a supportive community, you can find real change and peace. I highly recommend this book to anyone seeking a healthier, happier lifestyle.

JOEL WARSH, MD

Life Unbinged Food Plan Testimonials

from among thousands who have broken free from food addiction

For most of my adult life I struggled with food: what to eat, when to eat, how much to eat, how to stop eating. I had tried a number of different weight loss programs. Then God led me to Kristy and Life Unbinged. I realized my missing piece. She taught me the importance of surrendering this food walk to the Lord. I needed food boundaries AND Jesus. Life Unbinged is about much more than our weight and how we eat. This is about who we are and whose we are. I hope you will join us on the journey! —*Kerry-Ann*

This plan works! I was down 28 pounds in eight weeks and still dropping! Thank You, Jesus, and Life Unbinged! —*Rosemary*

I am SO glad that I took a leap of faith and joined Life Unbinged. I could not have anticipated all that I would learn when humbling myself before God and others, admitting this addiction, and trusting God to supply all my physical and emotional needs. I have lost 100 pounds in 11 months and am still going strong. —*Kelly*

This program truly changed my life! I had tried so many "diets" over the course of my life, but Life Unbinged is different! I now have tools to keep me on the path of health, wellness, peace, and trusting God! The plan is literally answered prayer! I am so grateful!!! Thank you. —*Carol*

Kristy could have easily lived out her freedom in peace and quiet with her family. Instead, she made the choice to allow God to use her for His glory, to see others set free. I discovered Kristy through her social media videos and I was extremely hesitant to start yet another diet program. I have a long history of diets and years of bondage to eating disorders. It's a miracle that I made it through. I didn't think I would ever be free. But Life Unbinged isn't another diet program. First and foremost, it's about seeking God and developing that most important relationship.

In practical ways, Kristy also teaches about maintaining food boundaries and what to do in the face of temptation. I've faced some extremely difficult personal situations and in the past, I would have used food to soothe and numb out. I still struggle but now I have the tools to get me through those moments. I've also lost weight!

Life Unbinged offers a high-quality, simple approach with effective teaching and assignments toward faith-based food freedom. —*Jennifer*

Life Unbinged is the easiest program I've ever done! I've lost 15 pounds quickly! —*Marissa*

My A1C blood sugar test result went from an astounding 11 to a 6.7 in just a few months with Life Unbinged. —*Teressa*

The Lord has blessed me and helped me release 32 pounds in two months! I am so thankful for finding the Life Unbinged program. —*Cindy*

I must share what God has done for me in the last 60 days. First is the grace He's sustained me with. More than enough to walk with me through the hardest moments of this journey. I have so much energy and a deepened thirst to continue to know Him more and more. I am free of food chatter and obsessive/intrusive thoughts all day! While my clothes are fitting much more comfortably, and the scale indicates my mass has decreased by 18.3 pounds, the true joy is in the freedom found in Christ through this program. Kristy McCammon, thank you for heeding the call of Christ to reach out to those who are still struggling. You're storing up treasures in heaven! To everyone on this journey—stay the course. Focus everything on Jesus and He WILL free you from bondage. This is my new way of life!! —*Katrina*

For the first time in my life I have hope that I can be free. I've learned so much through Kristy's example, compassion, grace, and gentle nudges. I'm a work in progress but I'm committed. I will always thank God for crossing my path with Kristy's. She and the Life Unbinged community are answers to many tears and prayers. Blessings! —*Jennifer*

Thank you again for blessing my life! I was in a pit of despair and misery. I had never felt more hopeless. Now I'm six months clean of sugar and flour. Six months free of bingeing. Six months of disciplined weighed and measured eating, three times a day. Six months of daily surrender. My head is in a completely different place. My heart is full of gratitude. AND the 50-pound weight loss is great too! You're a beautiful soul, Kristy McCammon. I see Jesus in you. —*Jamie*

I'm so grateful for this program! It was my missing link to long-term successful weight loss! Kristy McCammon has formed an excellent biblical course study (she has her degree in education and is a real teacher!). She walks you through the steps to surrender and the key to success in this journey to food freedom. I highly recommend the Life Unbinged program if you're struggling or need to solidify your path. It certainly worked for me!! I thank God for Kristy! —*Deb*

I've been eating with boundaries for the past five years. I'm thankful to say I'm at my lowest weight and fast approaching the maintenance phase. After trying all the plans, I know this is the one that works for me and the one God sent as an answer to my prayers. I'm part of Kristy's Surrender Sisters group and through that community, accountability, and having added the fifth boundary (staying connected to Jesus Christ), I'm finding the missing links. —*Tracy*

*life un*binged

life *un*binged

Faith-Filled *Freedom* from Food Obsession

Kristy McCammon

Taste and see that the Lord is good;
blessed is the one who takes refuge in Him.

(Psalm 34:8)

Table of Contents

PART 3 — Living Life Unbinged

PART 4 — True Freedom

Acknowledgements

Each and every person I've encountered along my journey to freedom helped to shape me. I'm grateful to so many people for their support and to those who encouraged and helped me create Life Unbinged and, ultimately, this book. Thank you.

In particular, I'd like to acknowledge the following:

First and foremost, I thank my Lord and Savior, Jesus Christ, for giving me life, loving me, and showing me the way to unlock the chains of food addiction.

Thank you to my husband, Shawn McCammon, who showed me unconditional love beyond what I knew existed. Thank you for loving me at every weight and size.

To my five children, thank you for letting me live life to the fullest. You all bless me every day and I'm honored to be your mom. You are the reason I wanted to break free to *live* the life I love.

To my son, who was particularly instrumental in encouraging me to share my story. I'll never forget the moment you said, "Just start sharing!" Then you put your words into action by helping me film my first YouTube video. I'm extremely grateful.

To my dear friends, Kerry-Ann and Katherine, you have been such a support to me personally and professionally. By listening, being a sounding board, helping me create ideas, praying with me and for me, being a support to Life Unbinged, and personally holding me accountable to an unbinged life, you have been a safe place for me. I love you both.

I appreciate every diet program and thank every fitness trainer and counselor I've ever worked with because, positive or negative, each encounter led me closer to the truth about my addiction and becoming the free individual I am today.

Thank you to my editor, Jen Miller, who provided countless hours of advice, encouragement, and guidance.

Dear Reader,

I'm so honored and excited that you've chosen to join me for this life-changing journey to freedom from food obsession. Welcome to *Life Unbinged*! Although the tone of this book is directed toward women, the transformative principles pertain equally to men who are battling food addiction.

My story may be similar to yours. I struggled with food obsession, overeating, and being overweight for most of my life. By 2017, in my mid-forties, I was at my most desperate. My weight had steadily increased and my food intake was increasing daily. I couldn't get my addiction under control. I had tried everything and I felt helpless and hopeless, not knowing what to do.

Beyond the physical and emotional weight I was carrying, I loved the life I was living. At that point, I had five amazing kids and a great marriage of twenty-nine years. I was working with my husband in his business, helping with my children's homeschool co-op, volunteering at church, and leading ministries. Yet a ravenous hole of fear was swallowing me. My food addiction was out of control. I was spiraling deeper into that darkness and I feared there was nothing else I could do to try to stop it.

I was scared that I would eat myself into an early grave and miss all that life had to offer.

While there was an extraordinarily joyful aspect of my life, there was that one aspect that was the complete opposite: food addiction. It was dark, terrifying, and out of control. I was spiraling emotionally, as though I were strapped into the pitch-black capsule of a frightening amusement park ride that never stopped.

On one hand was the *momentary* thrill of the ride—eating—and on the other was the truly frightening reality that I had no control. I was trapped, chained, held captive, and at the mercy of the acceleration and food's control over me.

That's how addiction often feels: thrilling in the moment and terrifying in the reality of imprisonment, chained, no control, and no keys to free myself. I was obsessed with food—how much I could eat, when I could eat it, how I could hide it, and how I could get more.

Like so many people, perhaps you, I needed real help, a way out, a plan, and the right keys to truly free me and keep me free from food addiction.

I kept researching plans and I tried every diet. I also read weight-loss books and journals, and I attempted multiple exercise programs. None of those unlocked my chains.

I was desperate.

Making matters more complicated, I falsely believed that if I just loved God enough as a devoted Christian, I wouldn't have this addiction to food. *Am I not praying hard enough? Why can't I have self-control?*

Eventually, I realized the issue wasn't even about food, nor about not praying hard enough. The problem was much bigger and deeper than diet, exercise, and self-control.

The problem was my *self-will* to eat *my* way. While that statement may seem obvious, I would learn much about the realities of self-will, eating my own way, and the principles put into action that are wholly transformative: the keys to freedom from food addiction, the keys to a life unbinged.

I had work to do from the inside out rather than the outside in—the opposite of all diet plans.

I needed to take a good look at God's desires for us and His extraordinarily plentiful provision of beautiful, delicious, and restorative food. And I needed to allow those bountiful gifts to take their rightful place in my life—with a practical plan. Our Father is the God of perfect plans. We simply need to understand the foods He created for us and the boundaries in His immeasurably expansive garden we get to freely enjoy every day for the rest of our earthly lives.

Following God's perfect plan of provision freed me from food addiction and the diet cycle. You'll see how as you move through the pages of this book. I lost 100 pounds and have kept it off for years now while *fully living life* at last and living out His best plan for my life.

He has big and exciting plans for you too, and being stuck in the cycle of shame, diet, weight loss, and any other addiction is not on His list! You can become free to live fully in His best. He offers only the best of the best for our physical bodies and our spiritual, mental, and emotional freedom, thriving, peace, fulfillment, and joy.

Let's back up a bit and talk about where the broken boundary of eating begins.

Many of us struggle with food obsession and addiction to processed sugar and flour foods. Many people have a propensity toward food addiction, which will emerge at some point in their lives. Mine began early in childhood. Incidents of childhood trauma and stressors put me in a position to use food for comfort, breaking the boundary of God's best for me. When a challenging event occurred, food was right there, offering temporary comfort, but ultimately, it led to physical and emotional discomfort, and I became chained in the bondage of addiction.

As I sought comfort in food as a young child, the boundaries of food were blurred. Food became my foremost friend and love for a long, long time, my closest companion for many years because I had learned early in life to *feed* my feelings rather than *feel* them. When feelings were even a little bit yucky, I didn't know what to do except eat through those feelings, stuffing them down. Every emotion and situation became a reason to turn to my friend food, and eat. My feelings were painful and food was a quick hit of temporary comfort. I call it a "hit" rather than a "fix" because those moments of temporary emotional pacifying with food are not true fixes (repair of what's broken). The hit was so compelling that I began to feed every emotion, not just fear. But fear led me to chain myself to food for every feeling.

- When you're happy, eat.
- When you're sad, eat.
- When you're mad, eat.
- When you're frustrated, eat.
- When you're excited, eat.
- When you're bored, eat.
- When you're celebrating, eat.

From early childhood, that broken boundary became the cycle of chaining and imprisoning myself. I was held hostage by food for four decades.

When I married my husband, I gained a homelife free from the stressors of my childhood, but not free from human emotions that life circumstances naturally continued to stir. Although I no longer had a reason to escape into food, eating was the response firmly linked to my every emotion. Eating was the only way I knew how to navigate my emotions. Eating all day was my learned management for feelings, and I was too entrenched and ensnared in that habit to free myself. Eating was the fundamental response in me where boundaries should have been. Consequently, food addiction drove me into mental, emotional, and physical desperation.

I had virtually flung myself over the cliff and was free-falling.

Increasingly desperate, I kept trying diets, every diet, with increasingly fading hope that I'd gain control and free myself from food obsession. I tried all the diets you've probably tried: Weight Watchers, Nutrisystem, Atkins, Slimfast, Optifast, Medifast, Intermittent Fasting, Low Calorie, Keto, South Beach, Grapefruit, Cabbage Soup, Juice Fasting, and Master Cleanse among many others. I also tried a variety of pills and supplements.

Nothing worked.

Of course there were temporary results. I'd reach a goal weight and stop dieting, but the food boundary was still in grave disrepair. So as soon as I'd stop a diet, the weight returned. I didn't know about food boundaries nor the other true and essential keys that would free me from addiction. That chain was far stronger than my will to stay on any human plan. I hadn't yet realized that the fundamental problem had nothing to do with food and everything to do with my heart. In addition, my demolished food boundaries and dysfunctional relationship with food kept me in bondage. I would come to understand exactly how God, with my willingness, could repair me, heal me, and set me free from food addiction—the core message detailed in this book.

I also went to a counselor and confronted her with determination. "I need you to solve my weight problem. I have everything else in order (my thought at that time), but I have a food problem and I need you to help me solve it."

She proceeded to talk about food and then said, "Food is the good girl's alcohol."

What? I was livid that she had just compared me to an alcoholic! I was the angriest I'd ever been in my life. My experience was that alcoholics' personalities changed when drinking. I viewed alcoholics as making poor choices. (I know, ironic.) I viewed alcoholics as mean and overall very aggressive. The effects of alcohol, in my experience, were very different from the effects of food. My thoughts screamed at the counselor, *How in the world can you compare me to an alcoholic?* My thinking was that there was *no* comparison.

Nonetheless, I finished that session but never returned. That was the end of that. I would have none of it.

Fast forward to today. I eventually came to understand that the heart and mind are drawn to food in the same way they're drawn to alcohol. Though the effects and outcomes of alcohol bingeing can be extremely different from food bingeing, they can share similarities: We become self-focused and irritable when we're food bingeing and consequently ignite this emotional chain reaction:

- feeling like perpetual diet failures
- feeling physically unwell, weakened, and less mobile by our weight
- feeling distressed by our excessive weight and the heavy chains of our addiction
- feeling guilt and shame for sneaky hoodlum behaviors, like secretly bingeing and craftily pulling an extra roll and brownie from the buffet or potluck table and slipping those into our purse or pocket

The ripple effects go on and on, not simply affecting ourselves but also those around us.

When we're unhappy with ourselves, we can easily project that darkness onto others.

We can acknowledge that food addiction, like alcohol addiction, draws our hearts into darkness, away from God and people, to serve ourselves. Addictions are escape routes from feeling our emotions and attending to our honest thoughts and feelings. Addictions will keep us stuck, chained, unhappy, and feeling unable or unwilling to do the hard work—heart work—because such work is difficult and uncomfortable.

As the common saying goes, "The only way out is through." And we're never alone on the journey when we're yoked with God and in supportive human relationships. We're not without the freeing keys, the healing directions, and the perfectly designed boundaries of restoration—each detailed in this book.

In *Life Unhinged,* I share how you can conquer your food addiction for good and how to do the hard work and heart work to prevent repeating the chaining cycle and stuffing your feelings.

Before I came to realize the answers, I despaired over the fact that food was literally everywhere I went—every playdate, potluck, holiday, birthday—every occasion. And since food is needed to live, my natural and well-honed thought pattern kept leading me back to my long-standing conclusion: *I guess I have to get on another diet—again.*

Frankly, I was tired of starting and failing diet plans. I needed to find the right and final solution. So I went to another counselor and announced, "I'm here for you to solve my food and weight problem."

"Okay," she replied. "Can we also talk about some other things?"

"No! *Food* is the problem and I want to solve it!"

"Will you trust me?" she pushed gently.

I had nowhere else to turn. I was desperate. So, of course, I said yes.

She asked, "Can we spend the next six weeks studying who God calls you?"

I bucked. "I already know who God calls me: I'm loved. I'm valued—"

"Do you live like that?" she probed.

Ah, the magic question. It stuck me and gave me pause. *Am I living like the woman God says I am?* No, I wasn't living like I was loved, valued, and treasured. I wasn't living like the woman God calls me. And I wondered how that tied into a food addiction solution.

After six weeks of in-depth study about my worth, we started talking about food. That was the day my life and addiction took a dramatic turn. I prayed desperately, "God, You have to deliver me! Take away my cravings and give me a new, renewed space for food."

That same day, I came across the concept of food boundaries.

I had to eat to live, but I didn't have to eat everything. And I certainly didn't have to eat all day long. I recognized that boundaries are beautiful indications of God's great love for us—His desire to protect us while lavishly providing the best foods for our enjoyment and health, just like in the Garden of Eden.

I began to view food differently, not only as a human need but also as God's bountiful, beautiful, vibrant, and perfect creation for us. In this book, I share "next right step" choices that are fulfilling for body, mind, emotions, and spirit. I share the right mindset and heart posture toward ourselves and food and exactly how your food boundaries can be restored, how you can become free from food addiction, and how you can be healed while enjoying God's great favor over you.

Because I had studied and understood the depth of my worth—who God calls me and you—I was more than willing to accept the plentiful gift of boundaries designed for my protection and greatest well-being. I realized I could live the rest of my life within the boundaries of the beautiful and vast garden. All the details are shared in this book.

My rescue boat had arrived, and I started paddling in the sparkling water of new possibilities and renewed hope that never ends. I've not looked back for another diet plan. I am free from food addiction and free to be fully me. I have freedom of heart and mind I didn't know was possible. The mental chatter of food is now quiet, I'm no longer food-obsessed, and I'm finally in a heart and mind place where food stays in its intended place. I eat three healthy and delicious meals every day and I live an abundant life in between. I've maintained that 100-pound weight loss since 2017.

Certainly, my journey hasn't been perfect; that's for sure. But we don't have perfection in this life in any regard. What we have is a powerful rescue boat in a glassy sea of grace and powerful tools that can unlock the chains of food addiction and keep us free—the heart of this book.

You can be freed from food addiction. Keep reading. You'll discover how to change your relationship with food and how to keep food in its rightful place.

Get in this rescue boat with me and the many others who have gained the keys to full freedom from food addiction. Together, you and I are going to write or rewrite our stories.

Let's get started!

Kristy

How to Use This Book

Life Unbinged is intended as a guide to help you to unlock the chains of food addiction and maintain your freedom for the rest of your life. Each chapter and assignment holds the keys. Completing each action step of writing (on the pages) and adopting the principles as your new and ongoing lifestyle practices are acts of turning those keys and unlocking the chains.

Handwriting in itself is an essential tool. Handwriting reinforces the importance of what you've read in the chapters and assignments. I encourage you to write freely in this book—notes, questions, your thoughts, feelings, and aspirations, whatever you desire that will further motivate you to "take the next right steps" in your day-to-day life and the special occasions and circumstances when food is an even greater temptation.

I encourage you to take your time working your way through this book. Allow your thoughts to marinate in the principles and allow quality time to complete the activities and practice the key principles of each chapter.

You're on the right path!

Trust the process laid out in this book and break free.
Commit to engage throughout the entire journey.
In other words, don't give up.
This plan works when you're committed to work it.
Then you'll experience true transformation from the inside out.

PART 1

The Food Plan and Basics

CHAPTER 1

Stepping Into a Life Unbinged

The Basics

WHAT IS FOOD ADDICTION? According to one expert,

> Food addiction usually involves a person experiencing a loss of control
> over their eating habits. Many individuals with food addiction eat
> more food than they should for their body type and healthy size. . . .
> While you can be addicted to any food, most people who suffer from
> food addiction are addicted to "junk foods," also known as "highly
> palatable foods."[1]

I was eating excessively all the time, foods that made me feel good in the moment,
foods I could escape into and wrap myself up in, foods that tasted really good, high in
flavor and high in sugar.

I felt emotionally and physically sick. I was bloated, tired, and low in energy, and
despite those negative reactions, I continued to eat the feel-good foods.

My brain lights up like fireworks when I eat processed foods, sugar, or flour. My brain
says, "It's go time. Let's go now!"

I can confidently say I was a food addict.

I'll be honest with you; the first time I said, "I'm a food addict" was very, very hard. I didn't want to say it or admit it—not even to myself. I didn't believe I was truly a food addict, but then I began to recognize that truth, and when I exposed the truth to light, that's the moment my life took a turn toward lasting change.

Let's look at what God our loving Father says about food:

> Whether you eat or drink or whatever you do, do it for the glory of
> God. (1 Corinthians 10:31)

I was not eating for the glory of God. I was eating to please and satisfy my desires, bringing glory to me, not God.

Because He loves us so deeply, wanting His very best for us, He calls us to eat in a way that brings Him glory as our good, good Father.

I had to ask myself how I would eat if my heavenly Father were sitting across the table with me. The answer was clear. Certainly not the way I would eat in private. I definitely wouldn't gather foods for a binge itinerary. Definitely not!

The thing is, He's always with us; His Spirit lives in our bodies, which He masterfully created and asked us to treat like His holy temple (1 Corinthians 6:19–20).

I was struggling to control my food intake, doing everything in my power to control myself, which had never worked. Then I realized God could do more with my surrender than I could do with my human control. Because I'm not perfect, never will be—nor will anyone this side of heaven—I needed God's help to fulfill His best for me.

My problem, from childhood forward, was trying to do life and make changes using my own limited strength. I was continually coming up with new plans, new diets, new exercises, and new supplements, but everything I tried failed. I came to realize that I couldn't change on my own. This profound understanding placed me at God's feet, covered by His great love and grace. There, I remembered that God leaves nothing undone. He had already created the perfect plan and had all along been offering me His keys to unlock my chains and the iron door of addiction. I simply needed to trust Him, grasp hold of those keys, learn to use them, and fully give myself to Him. I needed to live within the boundaries of His incredibly vast and beautiful provisions, which He had created in the very beginning—the Garden of Eden. He was offering me everything I needed and could ever hope for, including fulfillment and freedom.

Only when I allowed God to help me fight the battle was His strength made perfect in my weakness, as He promised in 2 Corinthians 12:9. How awesome is that?!

Just as a loving parent will respond to their children's cries for help, God heard my cry to Him—"Oh my goodness, God, I'm weak. I'm a mess! Please help me. Be my strength"—

and He gave me His divine strength. This is why He said, "My yoke is easy and my burden is light" (Matthew 11:30). Relying on His strength means we're partnered with the One who brings His superpower—resurrection power—to the table. He harnesses Himself to us and bears the weight of our burdens.

Prior to that verse, He gave us an invitation: "Come to me, all you who are weary and burdened, and I will give you rest. Take my yoke upon you and learn from me, for I am gentle and humble in heart, and you will find rest for your souls" (Matthew 11:28–29).

I needed to know that He was going to help me fight this battle. So I stepped out in faith and allowed Him to be my strength.

> *Your good and loving heavenly Father*
> *will help you fight your battle.*

A little later, we'll talk more about perfectionism, but know right here and now that you will never be perfect in this lifetime. We must each throw off the enemy's deceitful and damning spirit of perfectionism or we'll continue trying to claw our way out of our dark holes only to continue slipping back down into those ditches. Eventually we will slide all the way to rock bottom and even to an early grave—which is exactly what the enemy wants for us. Instead, we can choose to focus on being overcomers through the power of God within us.

Let's lean into the fact that we'll never be perfect in this lifetime. By standing in truth and asking God for His strength, we immediately expose the enemy's lie to the ultra-powerful, healing light of God our Father. In His light and strength, we become "more than conquerors" (Romans 8:37), equipped to make strides forward, growing, learning, and becoming stronger.

You are not alone on this amazing road to surrender. God is always with you and for you, and so am I and other Surrender Sisters. We have Him and each other in every moment of frustration, struggle, and celebration. "A cord of three strands is not quickly broken" (Ecclesiastes 4:12).

The Life Unbinged Roadmap

Along the road to a life unbinged, we're going to learn, grow, and surrender together.

We'll learn the tools of surrender and enjoy daily activities that lead to the freed heart and mind of full surrender to the One who created us. God knows and loves us like no other and wants only the very best for us in every regard.

> Taste and see that the Lord is good; blessed is the one who takes refuge in him. (Psalm 34:8)

First, what is surrender? Laying our will and every burden at the Lord our Father's feet. How? Surrendering ourselves fully to God and the riches of His kingdom allows us to continually renew our minds. You'll learn to recognize and grab hold of your willful and negative thoughts and replace those with the truth of who God calls you, His beloved daughter.

You may be thinking as I did when my counselor suggested I study who God calls me. You may ask why we would spend time in that non-food, non-diet study when we already know what God calls us. The deeper question is this:

Have I let God's truths about me sink deep into my soul and wash me whole?

If we really understood the depth of God's love for us and our worth as His uniquely created daughters, we could embrace our true value and His redemption. We would start living differently. We would come alive and become vibrant, blossoming, and confident.

The journey to life unbinged is the journey to fully surrender to our Father, beginning with our minds. Along this road, you'll learn these transformative wonders:

- why food has been such a comfort
- how to turn to God instead of food
- how to truly surrender your all to God
- how to free yourself from an all-or-nothing mindset
- the beauty of food boundaries
- how to let go of perfectionism
- how to give yourself the *grace upon grace* that God gives you
- how to renew your mind
- how to live like you are loved, knowing you are
- how to *not* quench the Holy Spirit of God dwelling inside you
- what the enemy of your soul has devised against you
- why the enemy, the father of lies, wants to defeat you
- how to develop a plan to conquer temptations and cravings

Those learning points in action will ultimately allow you to

- get off and stay off the diet merry-go-round,
- lose excess weight,
- drop the shame associated with overeating,
- say goodbye to mental food chatter, and
- with true freedom, fully live out God's plan for your life.

And there's so much more! You're holding a comprehensive roadmap to guide you through your long sought-after transformation. We've all tried transformation from the outside in by monitoring what food and how much of it we put into our mouths, and that direction failed us. Now you're stepping onto the Truth Road with a one-direction roadmap that leads to lasting transformation: from the inside out! It would be fitting to refer to this road as the *freeway*—free from food addiction.

So let's go!

What Is Your Why?

Why are you searching to change your plan, your course, to do life differently? If you've explored your why before, perhaps this roadmap will help you see your why with fresh eyes and a fresh perspective.

My why and my reasons for desiring a change were many, but my biggest were to honor God with my food choices and fully live the life I love. Although I loved my family and activities, I was eating myself to death—and on an installment plan. Of course that wasn't my intention, but that's what was happening. Had I continued to eat through my days and obsess about food, I would have continued in the direction of cutting my life short by adverse health: physically, mentally, emotionally, and spiritually.

The time had come for me to learn how to lay my negative mindset at the feet of God, where health-sinking habits stop.

I had a lot of other big whys, like being alive to watch my kids grow up and have families of their own. Some of my basic whys included walking up and down my driveway, taking hikes, bending over to pick up something and easily tie my shoes, crossing my legs, and other normal, physical activities.

Your turn.

Action Step: My Whys

List them all.

My biggest whys:

_____

_____

_____

_____

My basic whys:

_____

_____

_____

_____

_____

_____

_____

_____

CHAPTER 2

The Five Food Boundaries

THE PLAN IS NOT *ONLY* ABOUT THE FOOD. But we must have a food plan that clears our brain fog, inflammation, cravings, and obsession and gets to the heart of the matter, boundaries.

Before we talk about the boundaries, we must talk about what's inside those beautiful boundaries: three meals a day of delicious, abundant, wonderful, colorful, healthy, nutritious food we get to enjoy. However, if you have a modified food plan or have to eat smaller amounts due to medical reasons—perhaps even bariatric surgery—daily eating the same quantity of food spread over four to five meals is okay too.

The key mindset with each meal is knowing

- you're honoring God with your food choices,
- your choices are a surrendered meal you get to enjoy, and
- the meal is going to satisfy you while providing exactly what you need.

Nothing more and nothing less.

Let's dive into the food plan!

This original plan started in the 1960s with Overeaters Anonymous and continued into the 1980s with Food Addicts Anonymous. The plan is used by many other programs designed to provide four main food boundaries to keep our minds clear and bellies satiated. The food plan has stood the test of time and simply works.

But Life Unbinged has a fifth boundary that's even more important than the physical food and portions—time with God. Surrendering ourselves, our food choices, and our portions to God is where true transformation happens, so we're putting this fifth boundary in first place.

The boundaries are as follows:

- daily time with God
- three meals a day
- measured portions
- no sugar
- no flour

Boundary 1: Daily Time with God

The foundational boundary is staying connected to God daily. I encourage you to have a mindset of "conversation" with Him.

- Read and study His Word (the Bible).
- Pray to Him.
- Worship Him as your Creator and Father.

To be our best as God's daughters, we need this intentional, daily time with Him.

A counselor once told me that the only way to recover from food addiction is to "worship recovery."

Wrong.

I can understand how one comes to that conclusion. In fact, I've seen many people go from idolizing food to idolizing boundaries and recovery.

Neither is good or right. If we're worshipping food and then switch to worshipping boundaries, we're in no better shape and we're missing the mark.

God alone is to be worshipped. He is the Creator of all things, and we must honor Him as the One seated at that highest place. It is our Father who makes all things possible (Matthew 19:26).

Maybe we're down a few pounds but still have a heart toward worshipping something or someone as though it were greater than God. To avoid this trap placed by the enemy of our souls, daily time with God is essential. We must take time in God's Word, in prayer, and in worshipping Him to ensure that our mindset about Him and His provision of wonderful foods remain in their rightful places: God in the highest place and food in the secondary place.

Boundary 2: Three Meals a Day

Three meals a day is ideal to keep our blood sugar steady and our hunger at bay. In fact, once you've been on the plan for a short time, you may feel a little hungry right before each meal, but not the insatiable hunger and craving for more, more, more. Those feelings will have been replaced with normal, healthy hunger that's satisfied by our beautifully abundant meals. Three daily meals of delicious, abundant, wonderful, colorful, healthy, nutritious food. That's the beautiful gift inside the boundaries.

God gave us such wonderful foods. So it's important to focus on the food we have rather than the food we're not having, have given up, or don't want. Instead, we should rejoice over the beautiful, abundant food we get to eat each day.

We will look at specific foods and the food plan a bit later. Keep reading!

Boundary 3: Measured Portions and Meal Planning

Weighing and measuring food portions was not what I wanted to do when I first discovered food boundaries. Then I quickly remembered that what I'd been doing hadn't worked at all. What a small price to pay to know I'm getting exactly what my body needs each time I eat!

Determining specific portions also helps our brains avoid negotiating: *Maybe a little more of this. Did I have enough of that?* Then we argue with ourselves and can end up eating off-plan.

By weighing and measuring, the just-right serving is in front of you. Clear-cut, no calories, no macros—none of that. You're simply weighing and measuring your food.

Weighing and measuring makes the plan simple!

Choose a digital food scale of your liking. My favorite is the OXO Good Grips 11-pound scale with pull-out display. (See "Recommended Resources," page 212.)

If you want to take a scale with you to restaurants, potlucks, and other eating activities, there are portable scales that are very discreet.

Some people like to do a one-plate plan for different events and at restaurants. For instance, you know that dinner is one protein, one vegetable, and one fat, so choose your one plate accordingly. If you're at a buffet, serve yourself that one plate by carefully eyeballing the portion size. As you prepare your one-plate meals at home, measuring and weighing, you'll become better at eyeing portions.

Measuring and weighing precisely is important to help your body and brain know you're getting exactly enough—not too much or too little.

Preplanning your meals each day and writing that list for the day's meals will help you stay on track. I usually write my meal list each morning, before I eat breakfast. You may wish to write your list the night before. Either way, the point is that you're not dwelling on food throughout the day, thinking about plate possibilities. You have a plan laid out, it's lunchtime, and you already know what to grab. There are no dinner questions such as *What am I making?* You already know and you make that. Done.

I encourage you to write in a journal so you can look back at previous days. There are food journals on my website (www.lifeunbinged.com/store) or pick one up from the dollar store. What matters is *recording your food*, preferably ahead of time.

Here's the key thing to remember with each meal you've planned and sit down to eat:

I am honoring God with my food choices.

That knowledge and mindset is *surrendered meals*. A plate that will satisfy you with what you need. Nothing more and nothing less.

Boundaries 4 and 5: No Sugar and No Flour

Sugar and flour are ultra-processed powders and can be highly addictive. When we eat processed foods that contain sugar or flour, the powder immediately hits our bloodstream, turns into glucose, and raises our blood sugar. Because these foods are already broken down to the very essence, there is very little digestion that takes place. It gives us an immediate "hit" or "high." And when that "hit" is over, we are left wanting more.

An article published by the National Library of Medicine explains,

> "Food addiction" seems plausible because brain pathways that evolved to respond to natural rewards are also activated by addictive drugs. Sugar is noteworthy as a substance that releases opioids and dopamine and thus might be expected to have addictive potential.

> "Bingeing", "withdrawal", "craving" and cross-sensitization are . . . related to neurochemical changes in the brain that also occur with addictive drugs.[2]

Visualize this. If you put a large chunk of ice on the concrete in the sun, it will melt over an extended period of time. But if you shave it down and sprinkle ice chips out in the sun, they will melt almost immediately.

It's the same with wheat, almonds, oats, sugar cane, or any other food we eat. We can eat the whole, real food, and our bodies will break it down over time, giving us sustained energy and slowly releasing it to our bloodstream. But when we eat those same foods as ultra-processed powders, they become a detriment to our health.

God gave us all good foods to eat, packaged with water and fiber, because He knows what our bodies need. When we grind those foods into powder, we turn that blessing into a burden.

What about natural sweeteners?

Another way to think of the "no sugar" boundary is to think of it as a "no sweetener" boundary. Many foods like fruits, vegetables, and even milk have naturally occurring sugar that we will come to love and savor! However, it's essential to avoid adding anything to our food that would make it sweeter than it is naturally.

Although honey, maple syrup, dates, and dried fruit are healthier in terms of having minerals, antioxidants, and immune system support, the unfortunate truth is that they are too sweet for a brain and body that have been affected by addiction.

The sweet taste on our tongue is enough to activate the reward center of our brains and can trigger cravings and overeating. In my experience, it's just as easy to binge on cookies sweetened with honey and dried fruit as it is to binge on cookies made with processed white sugar.

The greatest freedom comes when we eliminate all sources of added sugar from our diet.

What about artificial sweeteners?

The food industry has marketed artificial sweeteners as a guilt-free substitute for sugar. For years, I drank diet soda daily, thinking that because it was calorie-free, I could indulge as much as I wanted and not worry about gaining weight. But it was just as addictive as regular soda and kept the sweet thoughts active all day long.

Many of us have that pull of artificial sweeteners. Whether they're "sugar-free" sodas, cookies, or ice cream, they are just as addictive and equally damaging to our health as sugar.

Research now supports the idea that artificial sweeteners do not help us lose weight and may even increase cravings and overeating.

Regular use of artificial sweeteners, even in the short term, can change our gut microbiome and make it harder for us to regulate our blood glucose levels, which can lead to other health complications.[3]

We will crave what we consume. Trying to give up sugar but continuing to consume artificially sweetened food and drinks, we'll never be completely free from the cravings and addictive pull of those foods.

To fight addiction and win, we must be willing to completely surrender all added sugar, sweeteners, and flour.

Tips and Tricks

Remove sugar- and flour-filled foods from your home (at least at the beginning of this journey).

If you have teenagers, they may sometimes bring in such foods, or perhaps your spouse likes to have certain foods on hand that are outside of your boundaries. In such cases, there are steps you can take to control what *you* choose to eat:

- Store those sugar- and flour-filled items out of your view.

- When others bring in such foods, respectfully ask them to hide them or store the items in a designated drawer or labeled tub with their name on it.

- Likewise, keep a tub in your pantry that's labeled with your no-sugar, no-flour foods. You don't want to run out of your favorites!

- Do whatever else is required to prepare yourself and keep your home a safe refuge from sugar- and flour-filled foods that tempt you.

- Ask your family members to hold you accountable. There are certain challenging foods that used to invite me to binge. When I bring any of those into the house for my family, I ask one of my kids to monitor the item, which may sound extreme, but if that support means keeping me *sugar sober*, I have to be willing to put that accountability in place. Advocating for ourselves is very important, so we'll talk about that a bit later.

- Don't stock up on items that were your binge foods. This is another beautiful guardrail! I used to struggle with eating white tortillas. Now, if I want to serve those with a particular meal, I only buy the amount I need for that one meal. That way, I'm not setting myself up to binge eat.

Important Reminder: Before starting any new plan for food, diet, or exercise, talk with your doctor or licensed dietician.

Three meals a day is ideal.

Meal Planner and Food Guide

3 Meals – Measured Portions – No Sugar – No Flour

3-Meal Plan		
Breakfast	**Lunch**	**Dinner**
1 Protein 1 Grain 1 Fruit	1 Protein 1 Fat 1 Fruit 6 oz. Vegetables *Optional Lunch* 10 oz. Vegetables	1 Protein 1 Fat 14 oz. Vegetables (8 oz. salad + 6 oz. cooked) *Optional Dinner* 10 oz. Vegetables

The "optional" noted is simply taking the 20 oz. of vegetables total and splitting it evenly between lunch and dinner.

Food Guide

Protein	Grain	Fruit	Vegetables
8 oz. milk (non-dairy too)	*Dry Weight: 1 oz., then cook*	*6 Ounces Total*	*Raw or cooked, weigh after cooking*
8 oz. yogurt	*Cooked Weight: 4 oz.*	berries	
8 oz. egg whites		cherries	*Example lunch or*
	4 oz. cooked millet	grapes	*dinner: 10 oz. total of*
6 oz. beans / lentils	4 oz. cooked polenta	mango	*any combination*
	4 oz. cooked quinoa	papaya	
4 oz. cottage cheese	4 oz. cooked rice	melon	artichoke
4 oz. cooked quinoa	4 oz. potato / sweet	pineapple	asparagus
4 oz. hummus	potato		beets
4 oz. ricotta		*3 Fruits*	beet greens
4 oz. beef	*(Cereals)*	apricot	bok choy
4 oz. chicken	4 oz. cooked Cream of	clementine	broccoli
4 oz. fish / shellfish	Wheat		brussels sprouts
4 oz. lamb	4 oz. cooked grits	*2 Fruits*	cabbage
4 oz. pork	1 oz. dry or 4 oz. cooked	kiwi	carrots
4 oz. turkey	oatmeal	persimmon	cauliflower
4 oz. shelled edamame	1 oz. Ezekiel cereal	plum	celery
4 oz. tempeh	1 oz. Fiber One cereal		collard greens
4 oz. tofu	1 oz. Uncle Sam's cereal	*1 Fruit*	cucumber
4 oz. veggie burger	1 oz. Shredded Wheat	apple	eggplant
	cereal	banana	green beans
2 eggs	1 oz. oat bran cereal or	grapefruit	jicama
2 oz. cheese	supplement	nectarine	kale
2 oz. roasted edamame	1 oz. quinoa flakes	orange	leeks
2 oz. nuts / nut butter		peach	lettuce
2 oz. seeds	*(Other)*	pear	mushrooms
2 oz. soy nuts	1 oz. rice cakes		onions
	1 oz. Triscuits		peppers
	1 piece Ezekiel bread		radicchio

	Fat	Condiments *(free foods)*	snap peas
	2 oz. avocado	8 oz. broth	snow peas
	2 oz. hummus	2 oz. plant-based milk	spaghetti squash
	2 oz. olives	2 oz. salsa	spinach
	1 oz. cheese	2 oz. marinara	Swiss chard
	1 oz. coconut cream	2 oz. ketchup	tomatoes
	1 oz. cream	2 oz. pickles	yellow squash
	1 oz. cream cheese	2 oz. pepperoncini	zucchini
	1 oz. sour cream	0.5 oz. nutritional yeast	
			Use Sparingly:
	0.5 oz. butter / margarine	*No serving size:*	acorn squash
	0.5 oz. dressing	capers	butternut squash
	0.5 oz. oil	cinnamon	corn
	0.5 oz. mayonnaise	herbs	parsnips
	0.5 oz. pesto	hot sauce	peas *(that are not listed*
	0.5 oz. tahini	lemon juice or wedge	*above)*
		lime juice or wedge	pumpkin
	(Other)	mustard	rutabaga
	0.5 oz. dried coconut	salt and pepper	turnips
	flakes	soy sauce	
	0.5 oz. nuts or nut butter	spices	
	0.5 oz. seeds	vinegar	

Modifications and Set Mealtimes

Some people, especially men, very tall women, and athletes, will need more protein. For these individuals, we suggest starting with 1.5 proteins per meal, monitoring weight loss, and making adjustments as necessary to stay within healthy limits.

If there are certain foods you don't eat for personal reasons or allergies, that's completely fine. Choose the items that work for you and consider trying new foods, condiments, and seasonings from the list. There are so many options, and the combinations are endless. The key is to honor God with your food plan and food choices.

As noted earlier, the Life Unbinged plan is designed for three meals per day. If you medically need four small meals or you're a two-meal-a-day individual for simplification or a longer period of fasting, set specific mealtimes, spaced apart (as no-eating times). (See "Recommended Resources," page 211.)

Eating is important for fuel and health. So commit to eating your daily pre-planned meal(s).

It is never a good idea to impulsively skip or add a meal.

Meal planning and commitment are key!

The food plan is just the beginning! With your plan in hand, the *heart* work begins. Please don't merely follow the plan and stop there. Keep walking through this book and applying the tools and principles as if your life and health depend on it. They do! There is freedom waiting on the other side.

Bonus Online Content

Free Colorful Eating Guide and Meal Planner

Action Step: Food Plan

1. Familiarize yourself with the food plan from God's gorgeous garden.

2. Practice writing a sample meal-planning day in the chart below.

3. Enjoy creating your new grocery list and give thanks! God loves you so much.

If grocery shopping in the aisles of the store is currently a temptation that feels too challenging, order online from your grocer and use their pickup or delivery service. The minimal fee will be worth it!

Sample meal-planning

Date:	
Breakfast	
Protein:	
Grain:	
Fruit:	
Lunch	
Protein:	
Fruit:	
Vegetable:	
Fat:	
Dinner	
Protein:	
Vegetable:	
Fat:	

CHAPTER 3

Preparing Yourself for Life Unbinged

Detox

WHEN YOU ELIMINATE SUGAR AND FLOUR FROM YOUR DIET, YOUR BODY WILL NATURALLY GO THROUGH A CHALLENGING PERIOD OF PHYSICAL AND EMOTIONAL DETOX THAT WILL ULTIMATELY BETTER YOUR HEALTH.

- **Physical detox** takes approximately five to seven days for most people. You may get headaches and feel tired and grumpy. While these challenges can be really hard, you can push through, knowing you're further freeing yourself from internal enemies. Your body will thank you later!

For those five to seven days, the key is to be kind to your body and mind, giving yourself an extra helping of grace. Rest, sleep, pray, embrace the emotional cleansing of crying, take baths, take walks, sweat, drink lots of water, and hold tight to this promise: "He gives strength to the weary and increases the power of the weak" (Isaiah 40:29).

With your diligent commitment in hand, with God's grace and strength, you will not only get through that week but also bask in the rewards of higher health and healing—more freedom than you can imagine! Your body, mind, and spirit will feel *great*!

- **Emotional detox** follows ridding your body of sugar and flour. After all, perhaps you've spent the last five, ten, twenty, or fifty years eating sugar and flour, stuffing your emotions, and feeding your feelings to not feel them. That's how I had lived life for so long.

The emotional detox was very hard for me. I wanted to eat. I wanted to just *eat* to shut down the yucky feelings. But I knew that the only way to get through the emotional detox was to allow myself to *feel my feelings*.

My emotional detox took approximately 30 days, and then I was in the groove of feeling my emotions. I spent a lot of time crying, grieving my relationship with food. That month was very hard for me because food had been my friend, my comfort, and my love for my entire life to that point.

Breaking free from that toxic relationship was one of the best choices I've made!

It's also important to acknowledge that the breakup was hard. I'm being honest with you to help you prepare yourself for your journey to further freedom. It will be difficult, but well worth the commitment of surrendering to God's best for you: literal new life in Him.

> Every good and perfect gift is from above, coming down from the Father of the heavenly lights. (James 1:17)

He has so much goodness for us, which is why He told us,

> Regarding your previous way of life, you put off your old self [completely discard your former nature], which is being corrupted through deceitful desires. (Ephesians 4:22 AMP)

> Blessed is the one who perseveres under trial because, having stood the test, that person will receive the crown of life that the Lord has promised to those who love him. (James 1:12)

But what's deceitful about our desires to overeat? The deceit is that food makes every trouble and every yucky feeling better. Deceit is from the enemy of our souls. Deceit is his name, and he will stop at nothing to woo us, then break us, keep us chained, steal "every good and perfect gift" (James 1:17)—like our joy, peace, and health—and destroy us.

Commit to defeating the enemy.

Put on the full armor of God because, during detox, you'll naturally have moments and situations the enemy will use to beg you to eat and stuff your feelings. When we get an anxious thought, that's the sign that he's summoning our "old self" to think, *I'll just eat.* Prepare yourself for that deceit and push through those moments. The enemy is counting on you to fall prey to every weakness, but you can stand firm, protected by the full armor of God.

You can get to the other side! Freedom is there and waiting, the immense reward that comes after pushing yourself through physical and emotional detox, breaking the chains of addiction.

There's no sugarcoating the truth here. After that first month, the hardest emotional part is over, but there's still grief. For years, you'll have emotions that will drive you to want to eat and times when you'll be tempted to return to your old self. So daily time with God (boundary one) is essential for guarding your mind against the enemy's traps.

Detoxing is not easy but always possible and completely worth it!

In the tough moments we must get through, we have God's promise: "My grace is sufficient for you, for my power is made perfect in weakness" (2 Corinthians 12:9). Rely on and rest in that truth, for "the truth will set you free" (John 8:32).

From Isolation to Involvement

Many food and sugar addicts (really any kind of addict) tend to isolate themselves when they're struggling. I did. We don't want someone to know when things are going badly and we're having a hard time. We just want to fix it and pretend like it never happened. That doesn't work and isolating is never a good idea.

We were designed for community to help and encourage each other.

We need community; we need each other; we need people. The enemy does his best work when we're in isolation because we're alone and we hear the internalized voices, the negativity. We feel the shame and guilt. So when you're tempted to isolate, DON'T! In moments of struggle, reach out and connect with others—not only for encouragement but also for sharpening. "As iron sharpens iron, so does one person sharpen another" (Proverbs 27:17).

Reach out to your trusted person, expose your thoughts and feelings to the light, and move forward without guilt or shame. Shame flourishes in silence. For these reasons and for daily encouragement, I urge you to follow Life Unbinged online:

- www.lifeunbinged.com
- www.facebook.com/lifeunbinged
- www.youtube.com/@lifeunbinged7371
- www.instagram.com/lifeunbinged

Ditch the Scale

Not the food scale, the body scale.

Not only do we have a dysfunctional relationship with food but typically with the body scale too. We allow it to tell us not only our weight but also our worth. A body scale is deceitful when we stand on it to see how we're doing or what kind of day we're going to have and what we're going to wear. Rather than a body scale being a weight mechanism, we allow it to morph into a control tower over us. Our quest for a life unbinged should be self-controlled and free from guilt, shame, and other negative thoughts about our beautifully created selves.

Body weight doesn't actually determine how we're doing or what kind of day we'll have. It doesn't get to determine what we'll wear or how we'll think, and it sure as heck can't determine our worth!

Break free from that deceitful, dictating relationship. It's been too complicated for far too long.

I recommend weighing yourself only once a month, if you can wait those four weeks. For some, it's hard to wait a month to see what's happened with that number. If that's the case, start with a more manageable waiting period—every ten days or once a week at the most.

Don't get on the scale more than once a week.
Do practice extending the waiting time.

If you're weighing yourself weekly, pick one day of the week, prepare yourself mentally (think "renewed mind"), and then step on the scale. Simply write down the number and move on. If need be, ask someone you trust to hide your scale so you're not tempted to weigh yourself every day. Ask them to get it out only once a week.

Weight cannot be the only number we use to determine how we're doing. Too often when we step on the scale and weigh less than we expected, we're more vulnerable to thinking we can let up a little bit and eat a little more. When the number is higher than we expected, we're more vulnerable to throw in the towel, say forget it, and ask ourselves in defeat, *Why am I even doing what I'm doing?*

We do not want to allow the number on the scale to determine our next step. It's simply a number that fluctuates because of various factors: what we've eaten, how much salt we've had, the time of month, and the time of day. Those factors have carried too much weight in our brains. We need to step back from that controlling relationship and use the body scale for basic information—and it's not the only tool we'll use. We can gain information from how our clothes fit and from a tape measure. But use those tools and the scale *for information only.*

Trust me, you do not want to let the scale be your dictator. It does not determine your worth. A simple and effective tip is to attach a sticky note to your scale that reads, "The number doesn't determine my worth. Jesus does!"

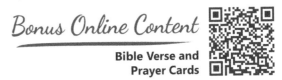

Bonus Online Content

Bible Verse and Prayer Cards

Temptation Plan

Whatever situation we're in, temptations will come. We live in a world where there will always be trouble, tribulation, trials, and temptation (John 16:33). It's just the way life works because we're fallible human beings. We must have a plan to squelch temptation.

Maybe you're at work, you've already eaten your compliant lunch (measured and free from sugar and flour), and someone brings out a tray of food.

What are you going to do? Are you going to look at it, think about the temptation, and ponder a decision?

Maybe you're at a party, facing a dessert table. Maybe you're at home by yourself and you want a second helping.

Those are the moments when we have to *pause.*

We must *practice the pause* to create enough head space to mentally walk through our temptation plan and make the next right choice. We're promised in 1 Corinthians 10:13 that no temptation can overtake us because God always makes a way out. But it's up to us to pause and find that way out.

At times, God will just deliver us, but like any good parent who wants their children to learn and mature, He most often allows us to practice overcoming our temptations. In doing so, we grow more mature spiritually, emotionally, and mentally. So we must have a plan to get out of tempting moments. Here's mine:

Stop, pray, and walk away.

That's also my favorite mantra.

When a dish is calling my name or I'm craving a certain food, I have to get myself out of the situation and get my eyes off the food so I can focus on making the better choice.

If I choose to stay in the tempting situation, pondering and fantasizing about the food, I'm very likely going to give in to the temptation. Instead, I choose to **stop, pray, and walk away!** This means that I physically stop my body, quickly ask God for help, and immediately remove myself from the temptation.

When I'm in a circumstance where I can slip away for a time, I go to the restroom or another private area, maybe outside, and I take five slow, deep breaths and pray.

Five deep breaths give us a solid stop to clear our minds and create the time and head space to make the next right decision, to pray.

When you're in a circumstance where you feel you must stay where you are, you can take those intentional breaths quietly, right then and there. Nobody has to see what you're doing, no need to be obvious about it. Right where you are, you can also close your eyes and talk to God from within, where the Holy Spirit lives, listens, hears, and speaks.

Then I reach out to one of my food boundary friends who also abstains from sugar and flour. Reaching out and saying I'm struggling exposes that truth to the light. I might even take a quick little video of myself saying something silly. Or I might have a one-minute dance party. Whatever action I take, I want it to draw me deeper into joy, gratitude, and connection. Addiction lies to us, telling us that the food will meet our needs, but when we stop, pray, and walk away, we're taking action steps of trust that God is ready and willing to give us something so much more!

> No temptation has overtaken you except what is common to mankind. And God is faithful; he will not let you be tempted beyond what you can bear. But when you are tempted, he will also provide a way out so that you can endure it. (1 Corinthians 10:13)

Action Step: Create Your Own Temptation Plan

Pick activities that will work best for your unique temptation plan, manageable steps you'll walk through BEFORE you reach for that food.

List the top five things you will do when tempted to eat something that's not on your food plan. Examples: stop, pray, walk away; take five deep breaths; call or text a friend; take a walk; journal; write a thank-you note; serve others; have a one-minute dance party; . . .

1. _____

2. _____

3. _____

4. _____

5. _____

CHAPTER 4

Truth vs. Lies: What God Says About You

Negative Thoughts

I USED TO LOOK IN THE MIRROR AND CALL MYSELF A LOSER. I would actually tell myself, "You're a loser."

When you look in the mirror, what negative thoughts, lies from the enemy, do you say to yourself? Or do you avoid the mirror as often as possible? Even then, what lies are recurring weeds in your mind? What thoughts run through your head when you step on that scale? How about when you put on a pair of pants? Even when our clothes are just a little too tight, most of us say very negative things to ourselves. I regularly said, "I'm never going to conquer this food issue."

So often, negative thoughts run through our heads. Maybe they're echoes of a bully's hard-hitting words from years past or the thoughtless words of a teacher or caregiver. Those negative words can haunt us years later and influence our thoughts and actions.

I had many childhood bullies in elementary school. Unfortunately, most commented on my weight. One was an adult—a teacher who said, "You're too fat to play. Go run laps." Those words still ring in my head at times.

One summer, I was playing with my kids at a waterpark, having the best time, when suddenly, a little thought skittered through my head. *You're too fat to play.*

No! I shooed the thought out and declared the truth. *No, I am not. I am worthy and redeemed and lovable.* Rebuking the negative and speaking the truth to myself was a new behavior. For most of my life, I had allowed such negative thoughts to stop me in my tracks and push me out of whatever I had wanted to do. Back then, I would have gotten out of the water, wrapped myself in a towel, subconsciously trying to hide, and sat quietly watching my kids play.

What negative thoughts run through your head—maybe from a childhood bully or teacher? Maybe a parent said some really nasty, mean things to you, intentionally or without forethought. Maybe your spouse has said negative things to you. Whatever the case, verbal punches and digs plow grooves into our brains, and we don't typically realize that we're carrying them forward, much less that they're influencing us.

Additionally, many of us have a running narrative we created against ourselves, a perpetual stream of poisonous thoughts in the background. Negative thoughts and patterns controlling our behaviors will continue until we recognize them and begin to intentionally renew our minds. Whatever the negative thoughts, we need to learn how to recognize them, practice staying aware of the sprouts, and pull those weeds out by the roots.

Jesus did far too much on the cross for us to think anything negative about ourselves.

God's Word speaks truth to us:

You are loved, worthy, and perfectly enough!

Renewing Your Mind

God also said we're redeemed and worth more than rubies. You're treasured and valuable. Maybe you already know that, but if you're like me, you need to let the truth sink deep into your heart, mind, and life.

Are you living like you believe all those truths about yourself? What can you do to allow those facts to change the negative way you think, make decisions, and live daily life?

I used to have a bookmark in my Bible that reminded me that I'm loved, valued, worthy, and enough. Although I believed those truths without question, I didn't truly reflect on how God sees me. I see my addiction behaviors as me floating on a raft in a pool of God's deep love and grace but never getting into that water of life. From my perspective, on my raft of addiction, I thought I knew how deep and how cool and refreshing the water was, but I had only floated on the surface.

It wasn't until I jumped in, leaving behind my addiction and completely surrendering to God, that I finally experienced how wide and deep His love is for me. Being fully submerged in God's love is immeasurably greater than and different from just floating on the surface.

Are you simply floating in trust that God loves you, or are you living in the depths of His love, experiencing that envelopment in every decision and having your daily life radically affected by His love and grace?

To win the war of addiction and live a full life, we need to live every moment fully submerged in God's love for us—moving freely in His love and seeing ourselves, our circumstances, and others through His all-encompassing love. Otherwise, simply floating on the surface, we're unable to fully see truth and experience God because we're exposed to surface chatter, the world's and our own:

> Girl, you're not lookin' good; you need those false eyelashes.
> You need to become a different size.
> You need this thing and that plan and these clothes to feel better about yourself.
> Your hair needs to be curled. Now your hair needs to be straight and a different color.
> Keep up with the trends. Get with the program.
> Trust us, we know what you need; we're the experts, the influencers.

The world will always tell us in countless ways and from countless sources that we're not enough.

Lies!

It's true that nothing we do from the world's view will ever be enough because it's all surface stuff that doesn't matter and because all people—even "experts" and "influencers"—are fallible. A vast majority of the world believes the lies rather than believing what our Maker, God, says.

> You are enough today, right now, and every moment hereafter. You are
>   perfectly imperfect,
>   perfectly beautiful,
>   perfectly redeemed,
>   perfectly loved,
>   perfectly purposed and gifted, and
>   perfectly being made new.

Not by a salon or a treatment or a trend, but by renewing your *mind* to continually think as God thinks. You are enough at your exact weight in this moment and the next, your exact haircut and style that feels good to *you*, and in the clothes you're wearing. If you've been wearing the same hairstyle for ten years and it feels right for *you*, good for you! The point is being enveloped *in* Christ rather than being a product *of* the world.

Jesus prayed to the Father, "They are not of the world, even as I am not of it. Sanctify them by the truth; your word is truth" (John 17:16–17).

Just as you are, created in God's image, you are sanctified (set apart, consecrated, holy) by truth. He said, "Let us make mankind in our image, in our likeness. . . . So God created mankind in his own image, . . . blessed them, . . . And it was so. . . . God saw all that he had made, and it was very good" (Genesis 1:26–31).

Very good. Wholly worthy, redeemed, and loved by the One who created you with perfect mastery. You and I cannot do one thing to enhance what God masterfully, perfectly created.

So, looking at the world, do you see why it's critical that we keep ourselves submerged in the truth of God's mastery—body, mind, and spirit? Only then can we fully live in the truth. How? "We take captive every thought to make it obedient to Christ" (2 Corinthians 10:5), constantly replacing every negative thought (lies of the enemy and the worldview under his influence) with God's truths about us.

When you live submerged in truth, you will feel worthy, redeemed, and loved, and you'll naturally live that way. Your life will open up like a cherry blossom in ways you presently don't know.

> ## *God called us into freedom—to live our daily lives in freedom of heart and mind.*

That's worth repeating: God has called *you*, _____, into freedom of heart and mind regarding every detail and aspect of your life. (Write your name on the line and reread the truth.)

Let's start right now, living every moment enveloped in the truth of God with a determined mindset to be transformed by renewing our minds.

Repeat the following truth of God throughout your days, for "the Lord's word is flawless; he shields all who take refuge in him" (Psalm 18:30).

I am loved, worthy, redeemed, and enough!

Action Step: Truth vs. Lies

Part 1: Lies

What lies do you hear in your head? What do you say to yourself? Do you call yourself a loser? Do you call yourself worthless? What do you say?

List all the negative words, phrases, and lies you tell yourself, those that other people have told you, and those you've otherwise heard and read.

_____   _____

_____   _____

_____   _____

_____   _____

_____   _____

_____   _____

_____   _____

_____   _____

_____   _____

Live life in practiced awareness of the voices in your head, taking captive every thought and exchanging for truth every thought that is not of God.

Part 2: Truth

Who does God say you are? What exactly does He say about you? Look up each Bible verse below and fill in the blanks, etching the truth into your heart. You're becoming transformed by renewing your mind!

I am God's . . .

John 1:12

_____

I have been . . .

2 Corinthians 5:17

_____

I have . . .

Romans 5:1–2

_____

I have been . . .

Colossians 2:9–10

_____

I can . . .

Philippians 4:13

_____

I am . . .

Romans 8:37

_____

I cannot be . . .

Romans 8:39

_____

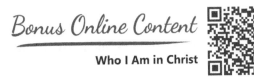

Bonus Online Content

Who I Am in Christ

CHAPTER 5

Live Like You Are Loved

SO OFTEN, WE LIST IN OUR HEADS THE THINGS WE WANT TO DO "WHEN I'VE REACHED MY GOAL WEIGHT" OR A CERTAIN CLOTHING SIZE. But the truth is, we can do countless things right now—most anything we desire, regardless of our size or the number on the scale.

The problem isn't weight and size. We allow inconsequential factors to hold us back from living a life we love (or could love) because we don't feel worthy.

Feeling ashamed, embarrassed, or unworthy comes from our enemy, Satan. "For our struggle is not against flesh and blood, but against . . . the powers of this dark world and against the spiritual forces of evil in the heavenly realms" (Ephesians 6:12). Thereby, living like we're loved and worthy must come from a mindset of *determined faith*, part of renewing our minds. The truth is that we don't have to wait until we're a certain size, or any other worldly-rooted factor, because we're already, right now, the individuals God loves—just as we are today and will be in all our designated tomorrows.

Of course, there are some activities we can't physically manage at various sizes and stages, but that factor is no different from the child who is three feet tall and thereby, for safety reasons, isn't yet permitted to ride the big roller coaster. Other examples are the high school quarterback who's not yet skilled enough for the NFL draft and the young mom who's not yet free to return to her former three-mile walk in blessed solitude.

It's perfectly okay and normal to move through life in stages.

Nothing of your time and experiences is wasted! There's growth in the uncomfortable, the disappointments, and the waiting. So why not live each day rooted firmly in the belief that you are loved? Why not do the things you enjoy, regardless of your physical size and any other factors?

If I say to myself, "I'm going to buy that piece of jewelry when I'm down to my next weight goal," or "I'm going to get that manicure when I've lost 20 pounds or fit into my new jeans," what I'm really doing is punishing myself. The enemy is highly skilled at dressing up self-punishment to look like a reward. Self-punishment feeds his lie that we're not *worthy* of a new item or joyful experience until we're—let's just say it—perfect.

Self-punishment is the opposite of what Christ said He came to give us. "I have come that they may have life, and have it in all its fullness" (John 10:10 BSB).

Live life now in all its fullness!

Self-punishment is like wrapping yourself in chains, from head to toe, all while Jesus is repeating to you, "I came that you, _____, may have life *in all its fullness*."
(write your name)

He already set us free. So why do we keep picking up the chains He threw into the abyss when He said on the cross, "It is finished" (John 19:30), freeing us from the bondage of our sin? When we continue to shackle ourselves, we're, in essence, believing that His sacrifice and resurrection were not enough for us or not for us. We must continually renew our minds in belief of who God says we are and live every day *in all its fullness*. There are no conditions, no "until . . ." attached to God's love for us and all that He lavishes on us as His daughters.

> He withholds no good thing from those who walk with integrity.
> (Psalm 84:11 NASB)

Integrity (right living, even when no one's looking) has nothing whatsoever to do with physical weight, clothing size, or any other chain and padlock that binds or judges.

Live like you are free—because you are!

Close your eyes and imagine Jesus standing before you.
Watch as He unlocks the padlock of your heart and mind.
Feel Him gently unwrap the heavy chains you keep purchasing from the enemy.
Now see Him throw the chains into the abyss, removed from you
"as far as the east is from the west" (Psalm 103:12 NLT).
Gone for good.
See yourself fully free.

Sit in that vision for a while. Return to it every time your mind starts to take a turn toward the abyss.

Jesus promised that He has set us free—period—to live every moment of every day in all its fullness. The decision to believe Him and take mind-renewing steps that shield your thoughts from the chain seller (Satan) is your own choice and doesn't change the fact that Jesus already removed your sins (chains) on the cross. Stop returning to his camp and buying his lies—those remanufactured chains that he disguises to look like awards.

Believe Jesus! "If you hold to my teaching, you are really my disciples. Then you will know the truth, and the truth will set you free. . . . So, if the Son sets you free, you will be free indeed" (John 8:31–36).

Will you believe Him? Will you live each day proving through your actions that you believe Him? The action verb "renewing" is an ongoing process, a daily journey of choosing to live by faith and renewing your mind, which is why Jesus also said, "Continue to work out your salvation" (Philippians 2:12). Your salvation—being set free from your sins forever—is God's free gift to you by faith, not by works (Ephesians 2:8–9). It's up to each of us fallible stinkin' thinkers to keep working on believing Jesus and renewing our minds.

Because our tendency as human beings is to keep picking up those chains, the work of living authentically by faith as the fully loved and believing daughters of the King requires that we put chain-breaking tools into action:

- Stay in God's living Word daily. The Bible is the "bread of life" (John 6:35) and the only bread we need—flourless.

- Memorize His Word, stay in it, and eat it up, and you'll "taste and see that the Lord is good; blessed is the one who takes refuge in him" (Psalm 34:8).

- Be on your knees in prayer regularly—and in your car and your bed and your shower and at the grocery store and the vet, . . . an ongoing dialogue with the One who loves you fully and has fully set you "free indeed."

- Reach out for support and accountability that will turn you back to truth whenever your mind starts taking you toward the abyss.

You are free! Free to be filled with the Lord's peace and to live in all the fullness of His joy—today and every day.

Okay, I get how you may not *feel* like you're free—yet. You may still feel completely drawn to food, for example, as I was, but everything you commit to change about yourself, no matter what it is, begins with renewing your mind.

Transformation began in me when I made the intentional heart and mind decision to *start living like I'm loved* and freed from food addiction, from food obsession, and from those extra pounds. The determined, renewing mindset to no longer wear the chains of my addiction and exchange those for the joy of the Lord is a moment-by-moment, grace-by-grace decision of commitment.

> ### *The joy of the Lord is your strength.*
> (Nehemiah 8:10)

A Thief of Joy: Comparing Ourselves to Others

We've trained our brains from an early age to compare. It's a well-rooted habit that perpetually calls to us: *Let's compare numbers; let's compare who's doing better and looks better.* Whether comparing our bodies, jobs, skills, or life journeys, we're inviting the enemy to steal our joy (our strength) and happiness. The result, every single time, is either feeling inadequate or the temporary feel-good of pride.

For example, a woman with kids at home looks at a woman who doesn't and assumes she can control what foods come into her home. Likewise, a woman who lives alone or without children sees a woman with a family and assumes she must have good support and accountability. Because others have different circumstances, we tend to assume that their challenges must be easier. That is often not true—another lie the enemy uses to trap us.

Comparison is always a losing battle and a thief of joy.

One of my favorite Bible verses is Psalm 139:14, "I praise you, for I am fearfully and wonderfully made." The verse prior says, "You formed my inmost being; You knit me together in my mother's womb." We must shut down comparison and speak God's truth:

God gave me a unique journey, purpose, design, gifts, strengths, and weaknesses.

When comparison sneaks in, take those thoughts captive, turn to your Creator, and speak truth. Memorize Philippians 1:6 and say it every time your thoughts drift toward the enemy's camp to pick up the chains of comparison.

> He who began a good work in you *will* carry it on to completion until
> the day of Christ Jesus. (Philippians 1:6, author emphasis)

We also don't need to worry about the good work God is doing in someone else's life in comparison to ours. He's faithfully completing His work in your life. So your thoughts should be steadfast on that good work. Remember that you don't know what's going on in someone else's life—even if they're your closest friend. Only God knows.

Let's focus on our personal relationship with the Lord and our own uniquely beautiful, wonderful journey. Let's encourage each other, lift each other up in prayer, and in every situation, ask ourselves these questions from Galatians 1:10:

- Am I trying to win the approval of man or God?
- Am I trying to please others or please God?
- Who am I truly living for—myself, others, or God?

When God created humankind, He said His design was "very good." He's the only One whose approval and validation we should seek. I want to live for an audience of One— my loving heavenly Father. In doing so, I can stand confidently before Him, knowing that my decisions are based on pleasing and honoring Him alone.

Easier said than done, right? Part of the nature of comparing ourselves to others is pleasing others. I'm a veteran people pleaser who is being transformed; so, I'm aware of the challenges. But I'm also aware that a key to God's best is knowing, believing, and practicing God's best: the truth that I am unique and free to live life to the fullest with no reason to compare myself to others.

We can do this!

Action Step: My Goals

Part 1: Goal Weight Goals

List all the things you want to do when you reach your goal weight. Maybe it's buying a new top or getting a whole new wardrobe. Maybe it's climbing a particular mountain, or perhaps riding a roller coaster, or taking that trip you've always wanted. Whatever your desires, list them below.

_____

_____

_____

_____

_____

_____

_____

_____

_____

_____

Part 2: Do it!

1.   Look at your Goal Weight Goals.

2.   Choose one goal, circle it, and go ahead and do it today or this week. If it requires scheduling, get it planned and on the calendar.

3.   I chose to _____ and I did it on _____!

     (date)

4.   Share your "I did it!" with a supportive friend.

5.   Below, write the details of your did-it experience. Go deep and be honest. These questions may help:

     • How did you feel, and what thoughts were going through your mind as you studied your list and made your choice?
     • How did you feel once you made the choice and began to make plans?
     • What thoughts did you experience as you set out to accomplish your goals?
     • What thoughts and feelings did you have while doing it?
     • What were your thoughts and feelings afterward?

_____

_____

_____

_____

CHAPTER 6

Perfectionism

EXTENDING GRACE TO OURSELVES IS DEFINITELY EASIER WHEN WE DON'T MAKE MISTAKES OR FALL OFF-PLAN. But perfection isn't reality.

Part of being transformed by renewing our minds is surrendering the mindset of perfection and holding tightly to God with the mindset of His grace and power at work in us. By His power, we can move past mistakes and failures and through tough times without the added weight of guilt and shame. Those were nailed to the cross with our sin, and grace has since *rained* and *reigned* over us and our fallibilities.

> Very rarely will anyone die for a righteous person, though for a good person someone might possibly dare to die. But God demonstrates his own love for us in this: "While we were still sinners, Christ died for us." (Romans 5:7–8)

Yet many of us want to be perfect and pursue perfection. When we can't achieve that impossibility, we feel like failures. A common mindset among most food addicts (and other addicts) is *all or nothing*. The problem is that it's impossible for any of us to *do it all*, and very easy to *do nothing*. Regardless of what we do, who we are, or what resources we have, this truth stands:

Perfection is impossible for human beings!

Imagine having a flat tire. Instead of trying to repair it, you decide to puncture the other three tires as well. All or nothing. Does that mindset make sense? Of course not! But that's exactly what we're tempted to do when we eat something off-plan. We think,

It doesn't matter now. I might as well eat this and that and the other too. That mindset doesn't make sense. It's total self-sabotage.

**Allowing ourselves to move into illogical thinking
is exactly what the enemy is after.**

Let's think about the tire analogy logically. Here are the five steps we act on when we have a flat tire:

1. Stop the car.
2. Get out and look at the problem.
3. Evaluate what needs to happen to get back on the road.
4. Extend grace to ourselves and the situation.
5. Fix the tire and get back on the road.

We can apply those five steps—five graces—anytime we eat off-plan.

Did you know that the biblical meaning of the number five is grace?

When you're reaching for something sugary or flour-filled, rather than continuing to reach and then throwing in the towel and bingeing, use logic and practice these five graces:

1. Pause.
2. Step back mentally and gain perspective.
3. Evaluate what needs to happen—the next right steps.
4. Extend grace to yourself.
5. Get back on plan with gratitude to God for His grace.

After a fall, an important step is to identify exactly what tripped you up and when. Ask yourself the following questions:

- What circumstance or environment was I in?
- What time of day or night did I enter into that circumstance or environment?
- What was I doing and thinking prior to reaching for the unplanned food? What comfort did I need that cannot be found in food?
- What will I do differently in the future to prevent giving in to temptation?

Here's the truth: There will always be a temptation because we live in a fallen world and have a fallible nature. So this life and our choices will never, ever be perfect. That's exactly why we're under the amazing canopy of God's grace. Grace is not only over us and our imperfections but also over the beautiful road Jesus paved for our human journey.

Do we expect perfection from our children? When they make mistakes and willfully disobey, do we cast them aside or rain harsh punishment on them? Or do we lovingly correct them on their learning journey and expect future mistakes and failures?

Our heavenly Father does not expect perfection from His children! He expects our failures and also expects our human best at the stage we're in. He expects us to keep moving forward and learning, and He expects humility, obedience, and perseverance. He also expects us to honor Him. He made this promise: "My power is made perfect in weakness" (2 Corinthians 12:9).

When you accepted Jesus as Lord and Savior over your life—the One who freed you from all condemnation of sin past, present, and future—you entered into "new life," a new journey, a new aim: to "be transformed by the renewing of your mind" (Romans 12:2).

Embrace this journey of new life, putting off the old mindset of perfectionism and putting on the new mindset of grace, gratitude, and ongoing growth.

I'm really thankful that God doesn't use our standard of thinking. He shows us the way forward through our mistakes and willful sin. Even at our worst, He doesn't change. He has forgiven us and remains faithfully full of grace and love toward us.

We can choose—right now and in every circumstance—to accept our fallibility and rest in God's power made perfect in our weakness. Let the following be your new-life mindset and prayer:

> I am human, not perfect. God does not expect me to be perfect, but to do my best to stay yoked with Him and within His boundaries. Because of His great love and grace, I can move through this life journey of growth with total peace, joy, and gratitude that I am covered by His forgiveness, love, and grace. He is my help and always makes a way of escape from my temptation and through my struggles.
>
> *God, my Father, I choose to honor You each moment with my human best, to learn from my fallibilities, and to see those as true blessings of growth.*

Stay grounded in this grace and truth:

I am on a fantastic, amazing journey that will never be perfect but perfectly paved with grace.

Pride Feeds Our Fallibility

About a year after I eliminated sugar and flour from my eating (2017), I managed perfectly for nine months—not one sugar or flour mistake, not one bite off the plan.

I was proud of myself. I was proud to the point of inviting arrogance, though not intentionally. While I didn't feel arrogant, looking back I can see that ungodly pride was taking root in my heart. I realize I was lacking grace and understanding when I'd see that someone had fallen off the plan and I'd think, *They should just stick to the plan!*

It's easy to forget the harsh road you've traveled when your head has risen high above it—until you free-fall and crash into it.

I lacked grace for others and had somehow forgotten that none of us can be perfect and certainly not retain perfection. I had also forgotten that "Pride goes before destruction, a haughty spirit before a fall" (Proverbs 16:18).

Easter Sunday came with all the usual festivities. A lot of food is around during that season—sugar- and flour-filled treats, baskets, buffets, parties, and candy galore. We spent the morning at church, had lunch at a buffet, and then went on an Easter egg hunt. That evening, we had another big meal. And guess what? I'd done great the whole day! Not one blip, not one bite off-plan. I was right on track but growing puffier with pride.

I don't recall pausing in the day for a mental and spiritual rest and reset. The day had been especially busy and fun with my kids, extended family, friends, and all the festivities of celebrating Christ's resurrection. And I was also celebrating my addiction success.

Celebrating successes is not bad unless those thoughts are full of helium.

My husband and kids had gone to bed. Everyone was tucked in and asleep, and my thoughts skipped a beat, kind of like a pinprick to a helium balloon. I vividly remember sitting on the couch, looking at multiple Easter baskets a little too long and with justifying thoughts (an open invitation to the enemy). *That was a long day! One piece of candy won't hurt.* His lies flew in fast and furious, and I rose with all that hot air, just like Eve and Adam had.

"Come on," he urged. "You haven't had one of those things in a year. Look at you. You've done great! Just one and then go to bed."

True. I hadn't had a piece of candy in a year and I *had* done great. So I ate just one and went to bed a little puffier with pride. *I only ate one piece of candy!*

"See! You can do it; you can have just one."

Had that been my voice or Satan's? Both. We were in agreement that night.

The next day, "just one" was all I could think about. *Just one more.*

Again, I had just one. Then, of course, my thought was, *Well, I'm already off-plan, I've already messed up, so . . .*

I leaped over the cliff, eating this and that and the other and another. . . . I remember that day most vividly because I then became physically sick and uncomfortable, which fed my emotional and mental discomfort, disappointment, and discouragement. I swore not to have any more the next day. *I'll get myself back on track tomorrow.*

That one willful misstep on Easter night derailed me for five days.

I was devastated and miserable in every way, physically and emotionally. I had fallen hard from my lofty place, and I knew I needed God's help in every moment. Perfection is impossible, and pride sets us up for falls.

Although I got back on track and have continued to be successful, the journey has not been perfect, nor will it ever be in this life. This journey is tough and fraught with Satan's invitations and schemes and my very human weaknesses. There have been moments when I've overeaten or grabbed a snack with this thought: *Oh, I can just have this little extra protein.* Nope, that never works. I need Jesus every moment and times of rest and reset with Him every day.

Stick with Jesus and the plan!

God uses our stories of imperfection to remind us and others that we're human, and in our weakness, God's power is made perfect.

Surrendering your all to God is one of the most powerful acts of grace toward yourself.

- Surrender your perfectionism and pride.
- Surrender to the fact that you are imperfectly awesome and your Father is abounding in love and grace toward you.
- Surrender to the knowledge that He will supply *all* your needs and will supply a way of escape from every temptation.
- Surrender to the fact that regardless of your human nature, your loving Father sees you as great.

Surrender how you think about yourself, your struggles, and other people. We each falter and fail, but our Father remains faithfully good to us.

If you overeat or otherwise eat off-plan, use the acronym G.R.A.C.E. to help you identify what led you down the path to the ditch or over the cliff and help you get back to God as quickly as possible.

G — Go to God first and foremost.

Go to God first and often, remembering that you are His child and perfection is impossible. He knows your fallibility and His love for you never fails, even in your mistakes and willful sins. "If we confess our sins, he is faithful and just to forgive us of our sins and cleanse us from all unrighteousness" (John 1:9). Go to God in full surrender to His best and lay your burdens at His feet. He is your true safe place. "Taste and see that God is good; blessed is the one who takes refuge in him" (Psalm 34:8).

R — Receive grace and reject shame.

Jesus did far too much on the cross for you to walk around in shame and dismiss His grace. "There is now no condemnation for those who are in Christ Jesus" (Romans 8:1).

A — Assess your mistakes and sin to identify why you responded unfavorably.

Assess to learn how you can respond with grace the next time. Ask yourself the following questions and journal your answers. Writing is a powerful path builder in our brains, and the bonus is that we can reread our answers whenever we need.

- What caused me to reach for that bite?
- What was going on right before I ate off-plan?
- What was I feeling?
- Have I been planning my meals?
- Did I stop to use my Temptation Plan? (Chapter 3)
- What can I do differently next time?

C — Cling to the truth of your identity.

Mistakes and all, you are the daughter of the King of kings. Remind yourself of this truth as a boundary against becoming frustrated, feeling like a failure, and feeling shame and guilt, which lead to spiraling into the black pit of self-degradation. Hold fast to the truth of what God says about you: You are loved, treasured as the Father's daughter, a co-heir with Christ, more valuable than rubies, and more than a conqueror. Not *feeling* like a conqueror at times doesn't change the truth of God: "We are more than conquerors through him who loved us" (Romans 8:37). Cling to the truth of your identity in Christ Jesus.

E — Equip yourself and stay equipped at all times with these tools for life unbinged success:

- the whole armor of God
- your written meal plan
- your written Temptation Plan
- the list of boundaries
- the self-grace to reach out for support and connection
- the steel mindset to stand firm in your commitment to Christ and God's best, to stay within the boundaries, yoked with Christ, to take the next right step, and to live moment to moment moving forward in freedom

Remember, "It is for freedom that Christ has set us free. Stand firm, then, and do not let yourselves be burdened again by a yoke of slavery" (Galatians 5:1). Jesus said, "My yoke is easy, and my burden is light" (Matthew 11:30).

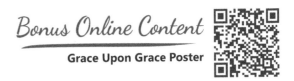

Bonus Online Content

Grace Upon Grace Poster

Doing It All vs. Surrendering to God

A mindset of trying to do it all is also a mindset of perfectionism—even if you know you can't do it all perfectly. Think about it. When we dig deeper, beneath the mindset of trying to do it all, we find the roots of pride and caring what others think about how we look, what we do, and how well we wear our many hats and spin all the plates.

We cannot be surrendered to God while surrendered to what others may think.

The world's gospel is the latest trends, fads, findings, and philosophies driven by media, influencers, and people around us. Time and again, we hear, "You can do it all! You can have it all!" Isn't that exactly how Satan tempted Jesus in the wilderness and Eve and Adam in the garden? He doesn't stop, but we can by surrendering our pride to Christ and caring only about what He thinks—our audience of One.

The apostle Paul wrote the following to believers. I've bolded key words and phrases:

I am astonished that you are so quickly deserting the **one** who called you to **live in the grace of Christ** and are turning to a different gospel—which is really no gospel at all. . . . Am I now trying to **win the approval of human beings, or of God**? Or am I trying to **please people**? If I were still trying to please people, I would not be a servant of Christ. (Galatians 1:6–7, 10, author emphasis)

Any part of ourselves and our lives that we place higher than God is an idol.

Jesus said, "No one can serve two masters. Either you will hate the one and love the other, or you will be devoted to the one and despise the other. You cannot serve both God and money" (Matthew 6:24)—money being an idol. "Those who cling to worthless idols turn away from God's love for them" (Jonah 2:8)—the opposite direction of seeking Him first in all things.

When pride is in play, our minds are focused more on doing it all and doing it all well—which is not a bad thing if we have an audience of One, our Heavenly Father.

We must ask ourselves this question: Who am I honestly trying to please as I'm doing it all?

- trying to stay godly and grace-filled
- trying to stay on plan
- trying to look my best
- trying to have the best
- trying to be the best wife, mom, friend, career woman, and volunteer at school, church, and in the community
- trying to be the best in my career while wearing all those hats

Who is the slave driver in me? I am.

Who keeps watering and wooing that in me? Satan and the world.

Who am I trying to please? Who is my audience?

Jesus testified by His *lifestyle* and *mindset* that God isn't a slave driver, nor is He waiting for us to mess up. That's the enemy's lifestyle and mindset! Jesus kept pointing people to His Father, our loving, compassionate, and jealous God who wants our full attention *so we can receive His best—the best of the best*. He wants our love and faithfulness and for us to give Him all glory, praise, honor, and thanks. He is the potter, and we are the clay (Isaiah 64:8). "Does the clay say to the potter, 'What are you making'" (Isaiah 45:9)? No. The clay is surrendered to the potter's will.

By our lifestyles and mindsets, we will lead others either to the world's stage or to the Creator of the world.

Jesus is our example; His audience was God. Jesus lived intentionally—slowly, orderly, and methodically. There was no racing from place to place. He didn't attempt to do it all and look good while He fulfilled His purpose. He certainly didn't follow the example of any human. Jesus traveled lightly with one goal: to bring glory to God—an audience of One—doing His Father's will.

> "I have come down from heaven not to do my will but to do the will of him who sent me." (John 6:38)

> Follow God's example, therefore, as dearly loved children. (Ephesians 5:1)

Our singular goal should be that of Jesus: fulfilling our purposes in humility and grace, bringing glory to the audience of One—God our Father. What does that look like?

- staying at Jesus's feet
- being proactive to seek Him first
- pursuing God and His purpose
- being persistent against the enemy and in doing our Father's will
- pausing to rest and recharge in His presence
- praying, studying, and memorizing His Word
- staying present and mindful of our thoughts, renewing our minds
- staying folded in God's grace, learning from mistakes and sin
- allowing our lifestyle and mindset to be the path that leads others to Christ

Let's rid ourselves of the notion of perfection, pride, and pleasing others, following the world, and pursuing everything that's billboarded along the dead-end highway of perfection. Pursue God and seek Him first in all decisions, desires, mistakes, failures, and struggles, and give Him all the glory and gratitude.

Action Step: Perfectionism and Pride

We're each different, but we all struggle in some areas with perfectionism and pride. What are yours? Freeing yourself from the chains of perfectionism and pride begins with honest confession of these before the Lord, in full surrender to His will and His ways, and also in giving Him glory for His goodness over you and in you.

Write your prayer of confession to God, specifying each chain of perfectionism and pride, and express praise, honor, glory, and gratitude to your Redeemer.

_____

_____

_____

_____

_____

_____

_____

_____

_____

_____

_____

_____

_____

PART 2

10 Tools of Surrender

This portion of the book is so very important that it warrants an introduction.

I would love to tell you that surrendering yourself to God's best for you in every regard is a one-and-done, like salvation, but it's not. Surrendering falls under that daily "work out your salvation" (Philippians 2:12) aspect of transformation I shared in Chapter 5.

Surrendering in itself is an ongoing process we must surrender to the Lord.

Surrender means laying our burdens at God's feet—giving them all to Him, including

- food obsession (of course),
- those flour and sugar foods we really love that became part of our emotionally insatiable hunger,
- our spirit of perfectionism, and
- the number on the scale.

Surrender isn't just a state of mind; surrender requires practical, tangible, day-to-day, meal-by-meal, craving-by-craving, and temptation-by-temptation actions that reinforce the surrendered state of mind. That mindset prompts us to make different choices from those we made in the past. Consistently making different choices—leaving our old selves behind (2 Corinthians 5:17)—is where we begin to see true inner and outer transformation.

Let's go through the surrender toolbox!

CHAPTER 7

Tool 1: Seek God First

LIVING FULLY SURRENDERED TO OUR HEAVENLY FATHER, WE'LL FIND THAT OUR GREATEST STRENGTH AND COMFORT ALWAYS BEGIN WITH SEEKING HIM FIRST, IN EVERY MOMENT AND IN ALL THINGS. This includes choosing Him and His perfect way instead of pleasuring ourselves with noncompliant food. As we practice seeking God first, minute by minute, hour by hour, day by day, surrendering becomes easier, more natural, and demolishes whatever we had placed higher than Him: our idols.

When food consumes our thoughts and actions, food is our idol.

I remember the times when I would come home from church, having a great day and feeling so connected with God, and I would want food. I'd have that feeling of obsession for foods I craved, pulling me from my seat at my heavenly Father's table. With that first thought of food, there also appears in our minds a dividing line of choice that we often don't pause to see and consider: God or gluttony. To choose the latter would, in essence, be saying to Him, *I'll be back; I'm just going to move away from You for a little while because I really want the food I desire.*

From as early as Adam and Eve—who were given carte blanche by God to eat of every tree except one—humankind has fallen for Satan's lies, perpetually turning to his ways first, which is exactly why we needed a Savior. Still, even though we know what

Christ paid on our behalf for freedom and fullness of joy, our sin nature gravitates toward anything and everything that's less than God's best. He doesn't offer or give us anything but *the best*; there is nothing on God's menu that's second-rate, yet we seek Him as an afterthought:

- in guilt and shame after overeating and bingeing
- in times we've deemed as obligatory: church attending, daily prayer and devotion, "saying grace" at mealtimes

So in our desire to truly be transformed by renewing our minds, the foremost question is this: What will I choose in this moment and every moment after? God and His best or my own way?

Every moment should be our starting place to seek God first.

Yes, it's hard to stay tuned to God in every moment and hard to surrender unhealthy habits, especially those pleasures we've held so dear for so very long. Both are intentional practices. Wouldn't we rather have God's best in every moment, His rewards, fullness of joy, and eternal pleasures by seeking Him first and doing the next right thing?

> You make known to me the path of life; you will fill me with joy in your presence, with eternal pleasures at your right hand. (Psalm 16:11)

Yes, there is some pain in surrendering our will and ways to God's, particularly at the beginning, when we're ending our clinging relationship with food. What breakup isn't painful?

Seeking God first and letting go in every moment, we gain so much more—His best, *the* best in each moment, plus His ultimate rewards: abundance in this life and throughout eternity.

As for daily life, Jesus asked us, "Is life not more than food and the body more than clothes?" (Matthew 6:25).

As for eternal life, He said, "Store up for yourselves treasures in heaven, where moths and vermin do not destroy, and where thieves do not break in and steal" (Matthew 6:20).

When we seek God first in every moment, in all things, we're safeguarding against the moths, vermin, and thieves of our self-centered choices that always leave us destroyed physically, mentally, emotionally, spiritually, and relationally.

God will never disappoint us because less than His best is simply not in His character. His gifts, His provisions, trump everything we could imagine. But to gain those, we must seek Him first.

When we want more of whatever temporarily satisfies, and even before we reach that point of gnawing desire, we must seek "Him who is able to do exceedingly abundantly above all that we ask or think, according to the power that works in us" (Ephesians 3:20 NKJV).

> "Why spend your money on food that does not give you strength? Why pay for food that does you no good? Listen to me, and you will eat what is good. You will enjoy the finest food. Come to me with your ears wide open. Listen, and you will find life." (Isaiah 55:2–3 NLT)

Lord, I'm listening. I choose You. I surrender what does not satisfy, and I delight in Your abundance. Help me use to the fullest capacity the tools of surrendering myself fully to You and receiving Your best for me.

Action Step: My Go-to-God Overview and Schedule

As I've shared, I'm visually oriented, so tools like the following overview and schedule are important for me. Seeing our lifestyles on paper can help us better renew our minds—in this case, our awareness of the time we seek God first. Creating a Go-to-God Schedule can help create an essential habit of relationship with Him and foster spiritual growth.

Important: The following overview is *not* meant to be shaming, guilt-inducing, or legalistic. The point is simply for you to see how frequently you typically seek God first.

1. Write down an overview of your present frequency in seeking God first.

	Day(s)	**Time Frame**
Church Attendance:	_____	_____
Dedicated Praying:	_____	_____
Reading and Studying God's Word:	_____	_____
Memorizing Scripture:	_____	_____
Worshipping:	_____	_____
_____	_____	_____
_____	_____	_____

2. Creating and following a Go-to-God Schedule will help train your thinking to be "God first"-centered.

Note: While prayer and worship should ideally become ongoing throughout your day—a *relationship* with God as your *companion*—setting specific times to be focused on prayer and worship is an essential starter step.

Again, this action step is *not* to create guilt or shame (enemy traps!) but to help you create and cultivate a deep, ongoing *relationship* with God and growing knowledge and understanding of Him and who you are in Christ Jesus.

As you're completing your ideal schedule, consider the transition times in your day, such as before meals, after work, the half hour before the kids burst through the door after school, before bed, early morning, . . .

Go-to-God Action	Day(s)	Time Frame
Church Attendance:	_____	_____
Dedicated Praying:	_____	_____
Reading and Studying God's Word:	_____	_____
Memorizing Scripture:	_____	_____
Worshipping:	_____	_____
_____	_____	_____
_____	_____	_____

Consider setting a reminder on your phone for each interval of action.

3. Perhaps make a photocopy of your Go-to-God Schedule to post on your fridge or pantry door as a reminder to be habitual in seeking God first.

CHAPTER 8

Tool 2:
Renew Your Mind

In Chapter 4, we talked about taking our thoughts captive (2 Corinthians 10:5) as the first step toward renewing our minds—exchanging old thoughts for new thoughts, which is like exchanging flour and sugar foods for new foods. If we're exchanging old thoughts for new thoughts, what new thoughts will fill us, satisfy us, and result in our contentment, joy, and peace? The answer is found in Philippians 4:8–9. Whenever a noncompliant food temptation enters our thoughts, whenever an ugly thought about ourselves and others rises, whenever guilt, shame, fear, and discouragement seep in, God says we are to think on these things:

- whatever is true
- whatever is noble
- whatever is right
- whatever is pure
- whatever is lovely
- whatever is admirable
- whatever is excellent
- whatever is praiseworthy
- whatever we have learned or received or heard from Jesus or seen in Him

His resulting promise to us? Peace. "The God of peace will be with you" (Philippians 4:9). The Lord "will keep in perfect peace those whose minds are steadfast, because they trust in you" (Isaiah 26:3).

The NIV offers the term "peace" to us 249 times and the word "joy" 242 times. My point? Clearly, God wants us to live in perpetual peace and joy. How? By perpetually seeking Him first, renewing our minds to think as He thinks, and trusting Him.

Look again at the above "whatever is" list. Each represents a countless number of good things for us to think about. For example,

- "Whatever is true": We've talked a lot about truth, such as feasting on who God says we are.

- "Whatever is lovely": This reminds me of a colorful salad, a gorgeous sunset, or the smile on a loved one's face.

Pause right now and reread the complete list. Beginning with "whatever is noble," consider the countless, wonderfully noble things God has given us to think about. Such thoughts are the ones that arm us against temptation.

When I'm thinking I'll just run through my favorite drive-through, I can instead choose to exchange that thought for "whatever is pure" and "whatever is praiseworthy."

Obsessive, negative thoughts can be triggered by images, like the brightly colored billboard of that saucy burger and seasoned fries. In those moments, I need to visualize what is pure and praiseworthy and engage my mind, heart, and actions in full surrender and seeking God first.

No matter where I am, I can take just a few minutes to renew my mind. If I am driving, I can even pull onto the side of the road with my hazard lights on (because my thoughts are in a hazardous place) and take five slow and deep breaths in prayer.

These breath prayers are a powerful way to engage heart, mind, and body—speaking aloud and visualizing the truth. With each inhale, say "Lord" (in your mind), because you've given your heart and life fully to Him. With each exhale, loudly verbalize praiseworthy truth.

Inhale and hold, saying in your heart:	Exhale and praise out loud:
Lord,	my body is Your holy temple. Thank You!
Lord,	You gave me a juicy steak I've planned to prepare and savor tonight. Thank You!
Lord,	You gave me a bin full of colorful veggies I've planned to enjoy. Thank You!
Lord,	what a table You've prepared for me! Thank You!
Lord,	You are my shepherd, so I shall not want. Today's compliant menu is amazing! Thank You!

Go ahead. Stop right now and give that practice a try. On the exhale, it's important to go all out—loud in praise. Don't hold back. Perhaps sing your praise as a new song to God or turn up the volume of your praise music. Either way, get your groove on and give all your mind, energy, and body to God in praise and worship.

> Sing to the Lord with grateful praise; make music to our God. (Psalm 147:7)

> Sing to the Lord a new song; sing to the Lord. (Psalm 96:1)

When we find ourselves fantasizing about food or simply thinking about noncompliant foods, we can choose to destroy those thoughts by renewing our minds with the mighty thoughts and images of "whatever is honorable, . . ."

- always leaving your willful thoughts at the feet of Jesus
- always taking confidence in the power of the Spirit of God within you
- always moving in the direction of God's best for you
- always seeking the rich bounty of His provisions and will for you

Continually renew your mind with pure and praiseworthy thoughts.

Practicing thoughts that are centered on the richness found in each "whatever is," we're guaranteed our Father's fullness of peace, contentment, joy, confidence, and more—all that we try and fail to gain and sustain in noncompliant foods, excess, and other hazardous habits.

Every action begins with a thought.

Reread that bolded fact. Let it be a marinade for your mind. Renewing your thoughts with praise and worship of the God of peace and provision can lead you to naturally and confidently do the next right thing: stay within the boundaries, in full surrender to God, and in His very best for you.

> He is my rock and my salvation; he is my fortress, I will not be shaken. My salvation and my honor depend on God; he is my mighty rock, my refuge. Trust in him at all times, you people; pour out your hearts to him, for God is our refuge. (Psalm 62:6–8)

Action Step: Read and Write Philippians 4:8–9

Write out Philippians 4:8-9 on the lines below.

Then write it again (or type it) on a notecard or paper and put it on your bathroom mirror. Read it daily and practice the renewing of your mind.

You can also put it on the refrigerator and recite it with others in your home.

_____

_____

_____

_____

_____

_____

_____

_____

_____

CHAPTER 9

Tool 3:
Practice a Posture of Surrender

Take a moment and think about how you feel when you're in an obsessive mindset about food and eating. That state of mind is a learned emotional protection that can morph into a feeling of desperation. That mindset is also a self-serving posture—*I gotta have that food hit!*

Addiction holds our thoughts captive:

- what I can get
- where I can get it
- how I can hide it

Maybe your hit looks like a quick binge in the pantry, out of sight, or leisurely sitting at the table in the darkness of night, or during the day when everyone's away, or in the bathroom stall at the office. There are so many ways we can find to hide and indulge our addictions.

This self-serving focus is our posture, not only the posture of the mind and spirit but also the body. Visualize your physical posture when you're obsessing, bingeing, eating in excess, and hiding the hazardous habits.

On the flip side, how do you feel and what is your physical posture when your mind and heart are set on doing the next right thing? Unhidden, head held high, looking upward to Christ, fully open to His goodness. Maybe your hands are reaching heavenward, and your mouth is praising the Lord as you feed from His righteousness, glory, and goodness. Perhaps you're dancing to God's singing over you (Zephaniah 3:17).

The posture of praising God and doing the next right thing is the posture of full surrender to His way and His will, which is very different from the posture of hiding and hoarding.

A surrendered posture says, "God, my hands and heart are fully open to You. Fill me with Your bounty—Your grace, mercy, love, peace, joy, and contentment—from Your table that You've prepared for me right in front of my enemies."

What a beautiful posture!

> You prepare a table before me in the presence of my enemies. You anoint my head with oil; my cup overflows. (Psalm 23:5)

> My mouth is filled with your praise, declaring your splendor all day long. (Psalm 71:8)

When my mouth is filled with praise, it can't be filled with cupcakes and chips.

One of my favorite quotes is by Holocaust survivor and author Corrie Ten Boom: "Hold everything loosely or else it hurts when God has to pry your fingers open"[4] (adaption).

The posture of loosely holding the things of this life, in full surrender to Christ, is actually part of my temptation attack plan for whenever I find myself thinking self-serving thoughts and envisioning food.

I love Merriam-Webster's definition of self-serving: "serving one's own interests often in disregard of the truth."[5]

Wow! I shared this twice prior but need to say it again: "The truth will set you free" (John 8:32).

Self-serving was the bondage of my lifestyle, the bondage posture of my mind and body for years. I needed a temptation attack plan against the most strategic of liars, the father of lies, Satan. "There is no truth in him. When he lies, he speaks his native language, for he is a liar and the father of lies" (John 8:44).

Down the road, maybe even today or tomorrow, you'll ponder a certain food that's not the best for you—a noncompliant food. In my times of mental battle, my hands are often clenched. *Oh, I want that food!*

In the first spark of thoughts that tempt you, **picture the dividing line of choices** that always appears, like this literal dividing line:

Do the next right thing: *praise posture* | Dive into the ditch: *self-serving posture*

That moment in time is not only the dividing moment but the *defining* moment.

- Will I take captive that food thought?
- Will I cast the thought at the feet of Jesus?
- Will I leave the thought at His feet?
- Will I immediately move my mind and body into the "whatever is" posture of God's will and goodness with praise to Him?

God promised to fill your hands, heart, and being with His sufficient grace, His great mercy, His peace beyond understanding, and "all comfort" (2 Corinthians 1:3). Each is far more filling than any food can ever satisfy.

Open your hands and heart wide and be filled by God.

- *Release* each self-serving thought to Jesus.
- *Trust* that He will fill your hands, mind, heart, and entire being.
- *Stay* attentive to your posture.
- *Feel* the difference between your surrendered posture and self-serving posture.
- *Stand* firm in your resolve to remain fully open.
- *Give* praise to God and dance before Him.

When I find myself clenching my hands in battle against my self-serving posture, I open my hands wide, whether in my lap or out in front of me or straight up, as if welcoming God and all of heaven into my hands. I don't have to make a big scene, but I do have to make a physically "open" posture change that reflects my thought posture: *I'm laying this self-serving thought at Your feet, Jesus. I need Your help and I praise You.*

Action Step: My Praise Posture

1. Describe your praise posture. If you don't yet have one, consider what that will look like for you and describe it.

_____

_____

_____

_____

_____

_____

_____

However long it takes for you to fully surrender into your unique praise posture, take that time.

We don't wait to practice fencing until the battle is upon us; we practice continuously to be ready when the enemy appears.

2. Right now, practice your praise posture, giving all of yourself to God.

3. Make this practice part of your lifestyle with Christ.

CHAPTER 10

Tool 4: Deny Yourself

DENYING OURSELVES ISN'T A POPULAR THOUGHT. Our world is centered on me, me, me as #1, foregoing the desire to become all God created us to be for His glory.

To deny ourselves is tough. Really tough, as with anything worthy. But this tool is essential to fully surrender ourselves to God and our need for transformation from the inside out. We deny ourselves to receive the riches of God's fullness waiting for us, including a life unbinged, a free heart and mind, and fulfillment that overflows. Hear this again and take it in:

We deny ourselves the fleeting things of this world to fully receive the riches of God that are waiting for us.

Denying ourselves doesn't mean no more fun; it simply means letting go of the worldly pleasures that are not God's very best for us—and certainly the harmful things like addiction and self-loathing. Denying yourself means surrendering fully to God—every aspect of your being and life.

Hear this: Do not swallow Satan's lies hook, line, and sinker, thinking that denying yourself is to live a boring, unfulfilling, legalistic, no-no-no life. What we're talking about as Tool 4 is denying ourselves the *few things* that are not on God's list of *best* for us among the countless good things He lavishes on us daily and calls "very good."

Let's revisit the Garden of Eden for a moment.

> God said, "I give you every seed-bearing plant on the face of the whole earth and every tree that has fruit with seed in it. They will be yours for food. . . . God saw all that he had made, and it was very good. . . . You are free to eat from any tree in the garden; but you must not eat from the tree of the knowledge of good and evil, for when you eat from it you will certainly die." (Genesis 1:29–31; 2:16–17)

Our focus must simply stay on the Lord's *very best* for us, for He is a good, good Father who gives good gifts *in abundance*.

> The Lord is my shepherd; I have all that I need. . . . You prepare a feast for me. . . . You honor me. . . . My cup overflows with blessings. (Psalm 23:1, 5 NLT)

Though "just say no" is not so easy, it's the next right thing whenever "this thing isn't good for me!" Whether the unhealthy pleasure is an absolute obvious *no-no* or a little thing that doesn't seem like such a big deal in the moment. "Yes, I could have this, but . . ." When there's a "but" whispering in your spirit, or screaming in you, ask yourself these simple questions:

- Will this pleasure benefit my walk with Christ and His temple (my body)?
- Will this pleasure delight God as I'm enjoying it?
- Will this pleasure brighten the light of God's glory shining from within me?

The world's answer to all desires is this: "If it feels good, do it! You should think of yourself first. Life is short, so live it up however you want, as long as you're not hurting someone else. Have it! Eat it! Smoke it! Drink it! Do it!"

But we—believers in Jesus Christ—are no longer our own (1 Corinthians 6:19–20). So when that unhealthy pleasure appears in your flourishing Garden of Eden, consider this too: If I were to strip away the "me, me, me," what would remain? The power and glory of the Holy Spirit, dwelling in my temporary temple of flesh.

The question then becomes: Will this pleasure be one that Jesus would enjoy?

> Put on the Lord Jesus Christ, and make no provision for the flesh, to gratify its desires. (Romans 13:14 ESV)

The NIV says it like this: "Clothe yourselves with the Lord Jesus Christ, and do not think about how to gratify the desires of the flesh"—the Holy Spirit at work in us from the inside out, filling us and fully clothing us and satisfying our every need.

Here's where we land as daughters of the King of kings, heirs to His throne, loved, honored, and lavished on by our Father:

We shouldn't even be thinking about how to gratify desires that are less than our Father's best—the desire to binge, overeat, hide, and ditch dive. . . .

The mind and heart posture of denying ourselves the yuck is an action of renewing our minds, grabbing thoughts that lead us to unhealthy actions, and exchanging those for what is healthy, whole, excellent, beautiful, and all the adjectives on the Philippians 4:8 "whatever is" list.

At the beginning of my journey to unbinge my life, I really struggled with learning how to eat well. Denying myself sugar and flour—the foods of bondage—and putting strict boundaries in place was difficult, to say the least. But denying myself the yuck became easier and easier, as does any new practiced habit. And for what? God's best, His Garden of Eden for me.

I can attest that denying yourself what is less than God's best will transform you to feel fabulous in every way.

We can do this!

Action Step: My Food Addiction Behaviors

With God's grace and goodness and our full surrender to Him in the safety of His arms, we can rid ourselves of the deepest roots of addiction behaviors, using the ten tools of surrender. Change begins with honest acknowledgment.

This assignment is not to create shame or guilt! This exercise is simply to help you start unraveling and peeling back the layers to reach the depth of your relationship with food versus the depth of your relationship with God. Climb into your Father's arms and trust Him as you do this deep gardening with Him.

1. As related to food and overeating, list every shame-inducing behavior you've done. You'll need to give this assignment some thorough thought to comprehensively complete. Again, honesty is key to becoming transformed and fully surrendered to God's best for you—fully free to enjoy the abundance of the beautiful garden He planted and designed for you.

    Through this exercise, you're digging up all the behaviors that have been ruling as idols and limiting your life. There's a litany of things we do when we're trying to get a quick hit for our addiction. My own list is long. In prior chapters, I've shared several of my own. Here are a few more common behaviors to help stir your memory of your own addiction behaviors: eating out of the trash, taking food from someone's plate when they stepped out of the room, and stealing food from other places.

    Again, take time to really dig through and dig up your addiction behaviors and habits from over the years, laying them all at Jesus's feet.

_____

_____

_____

_____

_____

_____

_____

_____

_____

_____

_____

_____

_____

_____

2. Having laid those before your loving Father, you may feel shame and guilt. But that's not His intention for you. Acknowledge each behavior to Him, one by one, through the following prayer, and receive His love, grace, and forgiveness with thanksgiving and gratitude, letting go of them and your shame and guilt.

_Lord, I _____. Here it is. Take it and give me Your strength to leave this at Your feet. Thank you for removing this and my shame and guilt as far as the east is from the west. Thank You for grace and love, Your power, strength, and goodness at work in me._

CHAPTER 11

Tool 5: Be Still and Know

GOD WANTS US TO REST AND TRUST IN HIM WITH THE FIRM KNOWLEDGE THAT HE IS OUR GOD. "Be still, and know that I am God" (Psalm 46:10). He knows we need this daily practice of sitting still before Him and pondering His sufficiency, might, and majesty. We don't have to have everything figured out. We can simply rest in Him and allow Him to hold us, carry us, and feed us.

I'm really big on visuals (if you haven't figured that out). Visualizing helps me be fully engaged. I can often picture someone trying to carry me when I've been injured or when I'm sick or overcome with exhaustion or grief. But when I'm fighting and resisting, kicking and screaming, scratching and climbing, that posture is because I'm prideful, thinking, *I've got this. I don't need help.* In that fighting and resisting posture, the person who wants to help me through my injury by carrying me and giving me rest is going to have a really hard time. We'll both end up getting hurt and bruised, and my destination will be delayed to boot.

Then I imagine myself surrendered and someone picking me up, putting their arms around me, and carrying me easily because of my surrendered posture. I envision wrapping my arms around their neck—a yoking together to make the journey easier and lighter—and resting my head on their shoulder. The journey forward will be much smoother, and I'm going to get the rest I need.

That is how I imagine myself in the arms of God—sometimes kicking and screaming when He's trying to carry me across a wickedly insane time. He always lets me choose my posture. "Be still and know that I am God" (Psalm 46:10) is not only an invitation but an instruction because He knows that the way forward will be far easier when I'm surrendered to Him carrying me. He explained His will and way like this:

> Come to me, all of you who are weary and carry heavy burdens, and I will give you rest. Take my yoke upon you. Let me teach you, because I am humble and gentle at heart, and you will find rest for your souls. For my yoke is easy to bear, and the burden I give you is light. (Matthew 11:28–30 NLT)

What does "yoke" even mean? He's not talking about eggs. He's using the example of an ox plowing a field alone versus two oxen yoked together—Him and you—making the work and the journey forward easier and lighter.

In all times—whether during temptations and trials, or successes and joys—our heavenly Father wants to partner with us and bear the load with us. He wants us to be in a posture of surrender—still and confident in His might. His strong arms and powerful love carry us through the deep waters, the parched wastelands, and the treacherous mountains of this life, which include the pitfalls of our own making.

He wants us to allow Him to pick us up. He wants us to wrap our arms around His neck and rest and trust Him in full surrender to His perfect will and ways, with confidence that He is the one and only true and living God.

Action Step: Be Still and Know

1. Take a moment to think about that stillness, knowing all the ways that God is *God*:

   - the Almighty
   - Creator of all things
   - timeless and true
   - living and present
   - faithful and unfailing
   - our help in times of trouble
   - our hope and encourager
   - our great physician and counselor
   - our loving and giving Father, who knows all things
   - the One who knit us together and gave us life, a purpose, hope, promises, provision, and more
   - the One who wants our full surrender and fellowship
   - the One who wants our all—our love, devotion, honor, obedience, and praise

2. Feel the power of your Father's invitation and instruction to be still before Him. Know and acknowledge His rightful place in your life, who He is, and who He says you are. Know that He is yours and you are His.

3. Set a timer for three minutes to practice this body, mind, and spirit posture of stillness and focus on God.

4. Now, write about your stillness experience. Be honest. After all, God knows all your thoughts and feelings. Your honesty will help free you as you make this time before God a daily habit. Perhaps these questions will help as you think deeply about your experience:

   - Did I stand, sit, kneel, lie down?
   - How did my position, stillness, and imagery feel, being in God's presence, knowing He is the Creator of all things, the all-knowing and all-mighty, the triune God, my Father?
   - Did I hear from God? What did I hear? How did His words make me feel?
   - Did I have any new discoveries about Him? What were they? How did they make me feel?

CHAPTER 12

Tool 6:
Practice a Spirit of Humility

WE CAN'T TRULY APPLY THE PREVIOUS TOOL WITHOUT A SPIRIT OF HUMILITY.

Imagine yourself determined to conquer your addiction. You're working hard, having some great successes on your own (without God's yoke), and you're proud when you have a win. Your mindset is, *I've got this!*

At some point—in the next hour, day, or month—when you're parading around proudly with 5 pounds less, the enemy will appear. You'll face a challenge that can drive you into the addiction ditch or over the cliff into the abyss of addiction darkness, shame, guilt, disappointment, discouragement, depression, doubt, . . .

Maybe the challenge will appear on Thanksgiving Day. Like a helium balloon, you're floating high on your pride of food-compliant success to date. Your mindset is, *I'm going to reward myself. After all, today is an extra-special food day.*

Enter: the family feast.

I'll have just one of those hot, puffy rolls with just one pat of butter. One ladle of gravy over one heap (I mean helping) of mashed potatoes won't hurt. And I'll have just one helping of Aunt Fanny's cranberry Jello-thingy dish; otherwise, she'll notice. Same with Mom's pie—she always works so hard to make our favorites and her grandkids' favorites for

Thanksgiving, Christmas, and birthdays. I'll have just one slice with only one scoop of ice cream. It's just today. I'm doin' so great living life unbinged! Today I can celebrate and feast with the whole family. Just today.

Exit: the trainwreck, powered by pride, crashing over the cliff into darkness. Not feeling so proud now. Not feeling so great in my body. Not feeling so great in my mind. And not feeling so great in my spirit.

Pride is a posture that leads to destruction. But God has made a way of escape from pride too.

"Humble yourselves before the Lord, and he will lift you up" (James 4:10) from the ditches and abyss. "He is patient with you, not wanting anyone to perish, but everyone to come to repentance" (2 Peter 3:9).

That image of Him lifting you up is the same image you carried through the lesson of Tool 5. Being still, surrendered, and humbled are three strands of a strong cord.

Action Step: Truths of Humility

Let's renew our minds with these truths about humility:

- Humility, practiced, produces the trust and confidence that "in all things God works for the good of those who love him, who have been called according to his purpose" (Romans 8:28) and that "I can do all things through Christ who gives me strength" (Philippians 4:13 BSB).

- Humility is a powerhouse gift of strength from God that we can choose (Proverbs 29:23).

- Humility is an act of trust in God to lead us through or carry us through, whichever is needed at any given time (Galatians 2:20).

- Humility reminds us that we can't maneuver well through this life and past every ditch and cliff without the strong arms of our Savior yoked to us. It also reminds us that we need Him and His yoke every second of every day to overcome and have lasting success (Matthew 11:30).

- Humility acknowledges that our way doesn't work nearly as well as God's and reminds us that His plan is always bigger and better and best (John 15:5).

- Humility keeps us open to the fact that a great temptation and a lot of little ones will certainly find us (1 Corinthians 10:13).

- Humility reminds us that we can "approach God's throne of grace with confidence, so that we may receive mercy and find grace to help us in our time of need" (Hebrews 4:16).

CHAPTER 13

Tool 7:

Connect to God: Scripture

FROM THE BEGINNING OF TIME, MEDITATING ON GOD'S WORD HAS ALWAYS BEEN HIS COMMISSION TO US.

> You shall meditate in it day and night, that you may observe to do according to all that is written in it. For then you will make your way prosperous, and then you will have good success. (Joshua 1:8 NKJV)

How do we know the commission is for us?

> Let the word of Christ dwell in you richly. (Colossians 3:16)

Can something dwell in us richly if we haven't ingested it?

> Blessed is the man [person] whose delight is in the law of the Lord, and who meditates on his law day and night. (Psalm 1:1–2)

> Everything that was written in the past was written to teach us, so that through the endurance taught in the Scriptures and the encouragement they provide we might have hope. (Romans 15:4)

> I have hidden your word in my heart that I might not sin against you. (Psalm 119:11)

Meditating on God's Word and memorizing it is pictured for us in this passage:

> These commandments that I give you today are to be on your hearts. Impress them on your children. Talk about them when you sit at home and when you walk along the road, when you lie down and when you get up. Tie them as symbols on your hands and bind them on your foreheads. Write them on the doorframes of your houses and on your gates. (Deuteronomy 6:4–9)

Meditating on God's Word is not simply reading it.

- Study the words and phrases, as well as the history and context.
- Study the true stories, parables, and prophecies.
- Study God's commands, laws, promises, and warnings.
- Ponder through the day what you've read and studied.
- Memorize what you've read and studied.

Meditating on God's Word is an intentional posture and process of your mind and heart, an intention to know, understand, and apply His Word in your daily life, in every circumstance.

> Do your best to present yourself to God as one approved, a worker who does not need to be ashamed and who correctly handles the word of truth. (2 Timothy 2:15)

We cannot correctly handle—live by or present to others—the Word of truth unless we're studying and memorizing God's Word. There are many Bible study helps, including Bible reading plans and apps. Best of all, we can pick up a physical Bible and devour it daily.

Don't be afraid to highlight verses and make notations in your Bible. The Word of God is "alive and active" (Hebrews 4:12), to be used fully in every way that will aid us in studying, understanding, and memorizing the Word. And what a heritage when future generations pick up your well-loved Bible and see your highlighting and notations leaping from the pages.

If you haven't read the Bible in a while, or ever, the book of John is a great place to start.

Also, pick up devotionals and study guides written by biblically sound authors. Supplemental materials do not replace reading and studying the Bible but offer explanations, practical thoughts, and prayers that will help you better understand and apply what you're reading in God's Word. Be careful not to place your faith in human authors, but test their thoughts by what the Word says in context.

Memorizing Scripture is a powerful tool of surrendering yourself to Christ. The beauty of studying and memorizing Scripture is that those verses and passages *will* come to your mind when you need them. And you'll be awed each time that happens. You'll feel and know more confidently that God is indeed with you and His Holy Spirit is communicating to you.

Other reasons we must stay in the Word, study it, and memorize it:

- The Word of God is Jesus. "He is the way and the truth and the life" (John 14:6). "In the beginning was the Word, and the Word was with God, and the Word was God" (John 1:1).

- The Word of God is the sword of the Lord against the enemy of our souls (Ephesians 6:17).

- The Word of God is nourishing food that strengthens our heart, mind, body, and relationships, conquers temptations, and allows us to be victorious in other forms of spiritual warfare as well (Matthew 4:4; 2 Peter 2:2).

- The Word of God is our solid direction, wisdom, knowledge, and plan for maneuvering through life with Christ, equipping and empowering us to renew our minds and do the next right thing (2 Timothy 3:16).

- The Word of God reminds us of our need for Him and our need to stay yoked with Him in order to be "overcomers," successfully facing and conquering with confidence and courage whatever situation arises in and around us (Romans 8:37; 13:31).

The list above is *not* comprehensive, for God's Word is limitless in knowledge, purpose, and power. We can present the Word of God (as I've attempted to do in this book), but we humans are highly restricted and fallible in what we can offer, for the Word of God cannot be fully attained by any one person except God, who is the Word. So for us to know the Word of God and memorize it is to

- *know Him* more fully—straight from God the Father, God the Son, and God the Spirit,

- *know how to* surrender ourselves fully to Him, and

- *know why* full surrender is paramount to attaining an abundant life, a life unbinged, eternal life, and leading others to the Life Giver.

Consider this: If you memorize one verse or brief passage each month, you'll have twelve engraved in your heart and mind by the end of the year. Then the next year, twenty-four; then forty-eight, and so forth. If you memorize one Scripture a week, that's a whopping fifty-two a year. Amazing!

Action Step: Read, Write, Memorize, Meditate

1. Choose a book of the Bible and daily read or listen to at least one chapter until you've completed that book. Then choose another book of the Bible and do the same, and so forth.

2. Make notes in a journal (or in your Bible), making special note of a verse or brief passage that God has drawn you to memorize.

3. Target memorizing one verse or brief passage each month. Perhaps you've read a verse I've shared in this book that you want to start with. The following is one of my very favorites in terms of my relationship with food and with God:

   > Taste and see that the Lord is good; blessed is the one who takes refuge in him. (Psalm 34:8)

Memorization Tips and Tools

- Whatever verse or passage you choose to memorize, read it again and again.
- Personalize the verse or passage by adding your name. Example:

  Kristy, taste and see that the Lord is good; blessed are you, Kristy, when you take refuge in Him.

- Take that personalization deeper by making it your prayer to God day after day as you're committing the verse(s) to memory. Example:

  Lord, I will taste and see that You are good. I am blessed when I take refuge in You.

- Meditate on specific keywords in the verse(s). Example—"refuge":

  I am truly blessed when I take refuge in my Father through prayer and His Word. In the past, I took refuge in food, the refrigerator, the pantry, and drive-throughs. Earthly things hold zero power of refuge. Only God can be my all-powerful help and shield, my fortress and strong tower in times of trouble.

- While various apps and other tools help us memorize God's Word, I encourage you to handwrite the verse(s) you're memorizing.

  Handwriting is scientifically proven to increase brain activity, which enhances our ability to memorize. Involving other physical activities during memorization will further increase that ability. Example: use dance or other full-body or limb movements while reciting your verse.

  Enhancing your handwritten verse by writing in cursive and on pretty paper or decorative note cards will also increase your ability to memorize.

- Post your handwritten verse on your refrigerator or mirror. Make a copy to post in your vehicle and another on your desk. Each month, exchange that posted verse with your new verse—but keep each written verse. You may want to display those in your bedroom or the hall on a decorated bulletin board. What a conversation starter and spiritual food for your guests and family!

*Taste and see that the Lord is good; blessed
is the one who takes refuge in him.*

(Psalm 34:8)

CHAPTER 14

Tool 8: Connect to God: Prayer

PRAYER IS SIMPLY TALKING TO GOD AS YOU WOULD A FRIEND, A FATHER, A COUNSELOR, OR ANOTHER TRUSTED PERSON. Jesus called Himself a friend. He is *the* best and closest friend, *the* greatest counselor, pastor, teacher, mentor, and healer—and He paid the cost for all our needs.

As with any conversation, there are different aspects and varying prayer times, but no rules. In Matthew 6:9–13, Jesus gave us an example of how we should pray:

> "Our Father in heaven,
> hallowed be your name,
> your kingdom come,
> your will be done,
>   on earth as it is in heaven.
> Give us today our daily bread.
> And forgive us our debts,
>   as we also have forgiven our debtors.
> And lead us not into temptation,
>   but deliver us from the evil one."

His prayer includes seven aspects, which is not surprising since the biblical meaning of the number seven is completion:

1. Acknowledge God as your Father.
2. Praise His name.
3. Affirm what He's doing on your behalf.
4. Surrender your will to His.
5. Ask for what you need (and desire).
6. Ask for forgiveness, remembering that all who receive Jesus as the one true Savior are receiving God's forgiveness.
7. Ask for God's leadership and His protection from temptation and from the enemy of your soul.

Whether you grew up praying or not, you may feel uncomfortable doing so now. So keep it simple and remember that you're speaking with the One who loves you fully and completely, as no human is capable. That fact in itself makes me want to crawl into His arms and talk with Him all day and even fall asleep in His arms while talking with Him.

Know this:

- Prayer becomes more natural the more you pray.
- No fanfare is needed.
- No special words are required.
- No particular time of day or length is set. Maybe you'll want to greet God first thing in the morning, talk to Him throughout the day, and fall asleep talking with Him.
- Even in silence, you can pray open-heartedly and honestly with your heavenly Father.
- Even in silence, singing to Him in your heart is a form of prayer.
- You can also write your prayers. You may wish to keep a prayer journal.
- Praying out loud or on the move (like a prayer walk) can be a powerful way to engage your heart, mind, and body.
- Foremost, just be yourself. After all, God knit you together in your mother's womb; He knows you like no other—even the number of hairs on your head (Matthew 10:30)—and when He created humankind in His image, He said it was "very good" (Genesis 1:31).

Maybe you're in the car, headed to an event. You can talk to the Lord.

Examples:

Lord, I'm headed to this event and I'm nervous. Help me. Thank You for always being with me and giving me Your power, strength, and peace.

Father, I'm headed to this event and I'm super excited. Woo-hoo! Thank You for this opportunity.

God, I'm headed to this event, but my kids are weighing heavy on my mind. I just don't know how best to respond to the issue our family is having. But You said You'd give me wisdom if I only asked. So I'm asking. And I'm believing that You're giving me the wisdom I need. Thank You, Lord. I love You and praise You.

Maybe you're on your knees, your hands clasped in a prayer pose because that feels a little more proper or reverent to you. That's perfectly fine with Him too. He is to be revered, for He is the most holy God.

No matter where you are or when, your divine Father wants to hear from you just like a parent wants to hear from their child. The difference is that God is always with you and will never leave you, but you can't see Him except through creation and in circumstances where you witness the work of His Spirit. His ears and heart are always open to you 24/7. He's eager to spend time with you throughout the days and evenings.

Prayer is a beautiful part of our relationship with Christ.

Action Step: Psalm 139

Dwell on your Father's love for you and His knowledge of you. Sit with Him in conversation, worship, and praise.

> You have searched me, Lord,
>   and you know me.
> You know when I sit and when I rise;
>   you perceive my thoughts from afar.
> You discern my going out and my lying down;
>   you are familiar with all my ways.
> Before a word is on my tongue
>   you, Lord, know it completely.
> You hem me in behind and before,
>   and you lay your hand upon me.
> Such knowledge is too wonderful for me,
>   too lofty for me to attain.
> Where can I go from your Spirit?
>   Where can I flee from your presence?
> If I go up to the heavens, you are there;
>   if I make my bed in the depths, you are there.
> If I rise on the wings of the dawn,
>   if I settle on the far side of the sea,
> even there your hand will guide me,
>   your right hand will hold me fast.
> If I say, "Surely the darkness will hide me
>   and the light become night around me,"
> even the darkness will not be dark to you;
>   the night will shine like the day,
>   for darkness is as light to you.
> For you created my inmost being;
>   you knit me together in my mother's womb.
> I praise you because I am fearfully and wonderfully made;
>   your works are wonderful,
>   I know that full well.
> My frame was not hidden from you
>   when I was made in the secret place,
>   when I was woven together in the depths of the earth.
> Your eyes saw my unformed body;
>   all the days ordained for me were written in your book
>   before one of them came to be.

How precious to me are your thoughts, God!
  How vast is the sum of them!
Were I to count them,
  they would outnumber the grains of sand—
  when I awake, I am still with you.
If only you, God, would slay the wicked!
  Away from me, you who are bloodthirsty!
They speak of you with evil intent;
  your adversaries misuse your name.
Do I not hate those who hate you, LORD,
  and abhor those who are in rebellion against you?
I have nothing but hatred for them;
  I count them my enemies.
Search me, God, and know my heart;
  test me and know my anxious thoughts.
See if there is any offensive way in me,
  and lead me in the way everlasting.

CHAPTER 15

Tool 9: Connect to Others: Iron Sharpens Iron

Proverbs 13:20 says, "He who walks with the wise will become wise, but the companion of fools will be destroyed."

Part of God's very best for us is walking life's road with other believers in Jesus. We learn and grow and are encouraged by each other's knowledge and experiences of the Word and life with Christ by sharing that life with each other. We can sharpen each other in our knowledge of God's Word just as iron sharpens iron.

The Collegiate Discipleship Maker published an article on this Hebrews 4:12 metaphor. Here is an excerpt:

> Ask anyone who works with knives, and they'll tell you that you're much more likely to cut yourself with a dull blade. More than that, cutting with a sharp blade is just a whole lot easier. Sharpness has value. It doesn't matter if it's a kitchen knife or a splitting axe or cavalry sword, a fine edge makes a difference. When the author of Hebrews wrote, "The word of God is sharper than any two-edged sword" (see Hebrews 4:12), he was making a point about the Bible, but he did it by equating its worth to sharpness.[6]

In the context of a life unbinged, and life in any regard, not one believer in Christ is without struggles. Most of us (if not everyone) have some type of addiction to varying degrees, and we're certainly all sinners. We need other believers as constants in our lives to lean on, to be a strong shoulder, to give and receive encouragement and accountability, to grow with, to mentor and be mentored by, with whom to enjoy the fullness of life, whether in times of worship, study, fun, laughter, tears, or celebration.

"Believers" aren't exclusive to those you know at your church and in your Bible study group. There are those who create Bible study books, audiobooks, podcasts, and videos of seasoned believers who "rightly divide the Word of truth" (2 Timothy 2:15). But there are also false teachers. Always be on guard for the enemy's schemes. Know and wear the full armor of God, and read and study the Word for yourself. The Holy Spirit is our greatest teacher. And yet, just as He provided Adam with a human connection with whom to share life, learn, and grow, He established His "church"—all believers in Jesus Christ.

How do we know which human teachers and authors we can trust to teach us the truth?

- First we seek God, asking Him to direct us to those who teach truth and asking Him for wisdom and discernment. James 1:5 says, "If any of you lacks wisdom, you should ask God, who gives generously to all without finding fault, and it will be given to you."

- Then step out in faith and ask believers you know—those who demonstrate a Christ-centered life with humility and knowledge—for their recommendations for Bible study tools produced by particular authors and online Bible teachers.

- Always, always, always compare to God's Word whatever you hear and read.

In addition, a very helpful connection place for those seeking to live life unbinged is our private online group of unbingeing and unbinged believers: Surrender Sisters, which you will hear more about toward the end of the book. We're dedicated to being in the Word, living the Word, sharing the Word, and discussing the Word. We share our struggles, offer our experiences, hold each other accountable, and yes, we laugh and have fun. This sisterhood is special because we're all working toward the same mindset and lifestyle: unbinged and living life to the fullest in complete surrender to Jesus.

> Let us consider how we may spur one another on toward love and good deeds, not giving up meeting together, as some are in the habit of doing, but encouraging one another—and all the more as you see the Day approaching. (Hebrews 10:24–25)

Action Step: Find Your Group and Bible Study Tools

If you're already connected with a group of believers, take time to pray for them. If you're not yet connected, I urge you to find your group and stay connected, no matter what.

Make a list of the people who draw you closer to Jesus.

_____

_____

_____

_____

_____

_____

_____

Now, plan to spend more time with these people. Iron sharpens iron.

CHAPTER 16

Tool 10: Remain Thankful and Grateful

THERE'S *ALWAYS* SOMETHING FOR WHICH TO BE THANKFUL AND GRATEFUL. What's the difference between the two? According to Merriam-Webster, a lot:

> *Thankful:* "conscious of benefit received."[7]

> *Grateful:* "appreciative of benefits received."[8]

If we're not conscious of what we have, we'll never reach gratitude. Remember Philippians 4:8? "Whatever is true, whatever is noble, . . ." describes an endless list of blessings and wonders. Seeking, finding, and listing the blessings and wonders in your life will help pave your path of boundaries with thankfulness and gratefulness. In your darkest days and seasons, a path cushioned with the specifics of God's goodness will bring you greater comfort, peace, encouragement, and motivation to do the next right thing.

Would I rather move through a dark tunnel on a rocky, unpaved, or worn road or a perpetually repaved (renewed) road?

God faithfully supplies all we need to maintain our road with thankfulness and gratefulness. We can thrive as we make our way through the dark tunnels to the other side of our food obsessions, addictions, and poor choices. But it's up to us to each look for all the blessings and wonders and keep a running list. Envision that list as your cushioned path.

Many of us have not understood the *why* of 1 Thessalonians 5:18: "Give thanks in all circumstances; for this is God's will for you in Christ Jesus." Even in the worst of the worst? Even when we don't understand why we have to suffer? Here are just a few thoughts.

Giving thanks in all circumstances generates these prompts and reminders:

- prompts us to find the silver linings
- prompts us to look for all that God has faithfully given and continues to give
- prompts us to seek Him for all our needs
- reminds us that He is what He says He is: gracious, faithful, loving, merciful, generous
- lifts our woeful spirits
- reminds us to continue standing firm on the eternal hope and promises we have in Jesus Christ
- reminds us that we are a light to others, reflecting God's glory that never fades

Foremost, we "give thanks in all things" because "in all things God works for the good of those who love him" (Romans 8:28).

Action Step: Living Thankful and Grateful

Keep a running list of God's blessings and wonders, and commit to adding at least one new one to your list every day, giving thanks and embracing that with gratitude.

Tips:

- There's an abundance of really neat gratitude journals, but a spiral notebook will do.

- When you're feeling that you can't find a different blessing or wonder to add, consider moving through your five senses:

  SEE
  > What do I see around me?

  HEAR
  > What do I hear near me and in the distance?

  SMELL
  > What do I smell? (Maybe you'll pick up on the detergent wafting from your shirt, or your deodorant. All blessings!)

  TOUCH
  > What do I feel by touch and in the air?

  TASTE
  > What do I taste within each item, this compliant meal on this beautiful plate? (Hint: sight bonus!)

Here's a fun alternative to a journal: Write each day's new thankful and grateful item on its own little card or slip of colorful paper and put it in a Mason jar or clear vase. Watch it fill up as your soul is daily filling up. That's another great conversation starter when you entertain guests, and certainly a beautiful example for those living with you. You may eventually find that you've begun a family tradition of noting the countless blessings you have for which to be thankful and grateful. What a legacy!

The thankful and grateful posture is not just about you (or me); it's about being the light of Jesus to others. He said, "You are the light of the world" (Matthew 5:14). In that context, He gives us some logic to help us remember His will. He said people don't "light a lamp and put it under a bowl. Instead, they put it on its stand, and it gives light to everyone in the house. In the same way, let your light shine before others, that they may see your good deeds [obedience to Christ] and glorify your Father in heaven" (Matthew 5:15–16, author addition).

If you're ever wondering what God's will is for your life, one thing is certain: You are to be a light of thankfulness and gratitude to God. You are also to

Rejoice always, pray continually, give thanks in all circumstances; for this is God's will for you in Christ Jesus.

(1 Thessalonians 5:16–18)

10 Tools of Surrender

1. Seek God First
2. Renew Your Mind
3. Practice a Posture of Surrender
4. Deny Yourself
5. Be Still and Know
6. Practice a Spirit of Humility
7. Connect to God: Scripture
8. Connect to God: Prayer
9. Connect to Others: Iron Sharpens Iron
10. Remain Thankful and Grateful

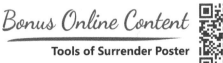

Bonus Online Content

Tools of Surrender Poster

PART 3

Living Life Unbinged

CHAPTER 17

Do The Next Right Thing—With Confidence

Have you ever heard, "just do the next right thing"? The concept sounds simple, but we've each experienced the strong draw of temptation that lands us in the food ditch, eating a snack, overeating at lunch, or giving in to a sugary treat.

The choice is always ours and the outcome—good or bad—is a testament to our commitment.

Either we'll stand strong and confident in our food compliance, doing the next right thing, or we'll take a detour into the ditch—eating off-plan and telling ourselves we'll start again tomorrow. Ditch-dipping is an indication of one or more of these signs:

- I'm not yet truly, fully committed to a life unbinged.

- I don't yet know how best to handle various food circumstances.

- I'm struggling with internal arguments or negative thought patterns and lack of self-control.

These and other issues that lead us to ditch food compliance can be conquered over time by consciously and consistently practicing the following commitment in every step of our day:

Do the next right thing.

The next right thing is the act of truth thinking and taking the best possible care of your body, God's temple. Doing the next right thing is a dedicated minute-by-minute commitment and practice. The journey won't be perfect, but day by day you'll grow stronger.

Going to God at each sight of a ditch (which Satan dresses as a delightful "dish") is always the next right thing. There's a ditch dish around every corner. So establish a go-to prayer of truth as God's way to help you escape. Example:

> Lord, I can *do* all *things—this next right thing—*
> *through Christ who strengthens me.*

When you're stuck in a moment, looking at the deceiving, delightful dish, such a prayer will remind you what God says about you: Your body is the temple of the Holy Spirit, who has already given you the power of almighty God, your victorious Warrior, to do the next right thing.

> I can do all things through Christ who gives me strength.
> (Philippians 4:13 BSB)

Don't look too far ahead; this battle is a step-by-step link of choices, like a stairway. Looking too far ahead, eyes on the destination, will cause you to miss the steps right in front of you, and you'll trip and fall every time.

> Yes, we plan ahead.
> Yes, we get a calendar and map out our plans.
> Yes, we buy our groceries ahead.
> But when we start moving through the plan, the bottom line that separates the ditch from the "I did it!" is *the next right step.*

One Day at a Time

We've also heard this slogan a lot, "One day at a time," especially in the addiction recovery world. In the food addicts' world, the mantra means there's enough to worry about today without taking on the added stress of what *could be* in the future. Jesus put it like this:

> "Seek the Kingdom of God above all else, and live righteously [right living], and he will give you everything you need. So don't worry about tomorrow, for tomorrow will bring its own worries. Today's trouble is enough for today." (Matthew 6:33–34 NLT, author addition)

Let's not worry about what restaurant we're going to or what will be served at a wedding or baby shower. Place your concern on the plate in front of you today (figuratively and literally) and simply plan for (instead of focusing on) what may be ahead.

Focus on winning today's battles with Christ's power in you.

How? Lay your food obsession at the feet of Jesus in every moment, and as you plan your meals, enjoy your meals, and when you encounter temptation, take the next right step. "We are more than conquerors through him who loved us" (Romans 8:37).

Today's focus is *today*, and each moment's focus is the next right step.

Confidence

Have you ever met someone with incredible confidence? Someone you can just tell is comfortable and confident in their own skin by the way they walk? It's common in the journey to a life unbinged to lack confidence in our ability to acclimate to boundaries and focus on the next right step. Thankfully, we don't have to rely on our own confidence, only on the confidence of knowing who we are in Christ—loved, valued, redeemed, purposed, and equipped. I'm talking about a totally radical confidence that *you can do anything* God puts on your heart to do—like this life unbinged. With a spirit of humility, knowing that such confidence is not in yourself but in the One who created you and called you by name, you *can* be wholly confident in each step!

> Blessed is the one who trusts in the Lord, whose confidence is in him.
> (Jeremiah 17:7)

Begin now to walk with confidence in Him that you are worthy of receiving and living life in God's very best. Take up confidence in Christ, who makes your path straight, equips you, and leads you in the way of righteousness that causes you to walk and move about your day differently—in confidence as a beloved daughter of the King of kings.

How to Advocate for Yourself

A tool God has given us to stand up against the enemy and stand confidently in our true worth is the ability to advocate for our needs and desires. You are worthy of speaking up for yourself. A number of Scripture verses point us to advocating for ourselves. Here are three:

> "Ask and it will be given to you; seek and you will find; knock and the door will be opened to you. For everyone who asks receives; the one who seeks finds; and to the one who knocks, the door will be opened."
> (Matthew 7:7)

We should come with boldness to the throne of grace, so that we may receive mercy and may find grace for help in time of need. (Hebrews 4:16 BLB)

In every situation, by prayer and petition, with thanksgiving, present your requests to God. (Philippians 4:6)

Many people I've spoken with, especially food addicts, addicts in general, and people pleasers, don't like to create waves by advocating for themselves. *I don't want to upset anybody. I don't want to offend anybody.* Consequently, many of my regretful decisions are because I didn't speak up for myself. Christ tells us to speak up for ourselves and to advocate for what is right. It's important for you to know that you are worthy to voice your needs—whether in a restaurant, in your home, or with a friend. You may not feel comfortable speaking up for yourself, but practicing this truth will help you gain confidence for any situation.

Let's say you're in a restaurant and need to order your salad without the croutons and the baked chicken without the sweet sauce. Are you comfortable speaking up for yourself?

Let's say you've specified your needs to the waiter, but when your meal arrives with croutons (i.e., flour) and sweet sauce (i.e., sugar), are you comfortable sending it back?

I must reiterate that advocating for yourself is essential. It gets easier every time, just as a muscle gets stronger each time you use it.

Speak up! You're worth advocating for your needs.

When I first started practicing the boundaries of avoiding sugar and flour, people around me weren't used to my change either. For example, a friend and I had spent a lot of time together overeating. We'd sit at a coffee shop and eat pastries and drink those sugar-heavy drinks. Well, about a week or two into my unbinged journey, she arrived at my house with a beautiful drink in hand, part of our past together. When I opened the door, she said, "Here you go!" I stood there (probably like a deer in headlights), not knowing what to do. I was in new territory too. *Do I drink it and then run the risk that I'm going to drink more later? Do I just take a sip? Or do I say I'm not feeling well? What am I going to do?*

In that moment of temptation, I realized that whatever decision I made would determine my future behaviors, including my courage to speak up.

I decided I wouldn't drink the gift. *But how do I say that to my friend?*

I simply said with kindness, "You know, I'm not having sugar right now because it's really been bothering me lately." I didn't have to go into a big spiel. I didn't have to say

I had cut out sugar and I'd never have that drink again. But I did have to advocate for myself as the next right step.

I could see she wanted me to drink her gift. However, I stuck to the best decision for my body, which helped to solidify my decisions from the beginning. Speaking up for myself was one of those decisions.

Becoming transformed takes time and advocacy, but we don't want to create waves, offend, or otherwise upset anyone. Yet courage is required to "lay aside the old self . . . and put on the new self" (Ephesians 4:22, 24 NASB1995). And we can choose to speak the truth in love (Ephesians 4:15).

Another example is when my mother-in-law made an amazing dessert for me. She knew about my boundaries and honestly thought the special recipe was something I could eat because it only contained bananas, eggs, and oats. Fair enough. She served it after Christmas dinner and said excitedly, "Here's the dessert I've made!" My father-in-law chimed in, "She's been searching for a recipe she could make for you, and she could hardly wait for you to try it."

I was again faced with a really hard decision. Even though the dessert was boundary-compliant—no sugar and no flour—I chose not to eat it for two other boundary reasons: I had not planned for that and had already eaten all my planned foods for the day. So there I was, wondering how to tell my excited and thoughtful loved one, who'd gone out of her way to prepare a special dessert with my needs in mind, that I couldn't eat it—without hurting her (and my father-in-law's) feelings.

I simply spoke the truth in love, genuinely touched. "Oh my gosh, that looks amazing! It sounds so great! I'm totally full right now. So do you mind if I take it home and eat it in the morning for breakfast?" I could then plan for the dish—a serious matter of my commitment to stick with the plan rather than eating impulsively.

They both said, "Of course," maybe a little put off that I didn't try a bite. But I'd advocated for what was best for me while doing my best to avoid hurting them.

Every challenge is a growth and strengthening opportunity.

The next morning, having planned for the compliant item, I enjoyed it for breakfast, took a picture, and sent it to them with my sincere thanks. I got to move through the day, and the previous one, with my head held high for standing up for my needs.

You must be willing to practice advocating for yourself—and today is the day to start! Speak up for your needs. If standing up for yourself is a struggle for you, know that each victory will strengthen you for the next, and little by little, you'll find that you've become comfortable and confident in doing so. I promise this renewal of your mind will be transformative and one of the best practices toward God's very best for you.

Action Step: Advocating for Myself

1. On the Life Unbinged confidence scale of one to five—1 being the least confident in advocating for yourself—where are you currently sitting? Be honest with yourself.

1   2   3   4   5

2. When you read "advocate for yourself," what image(s) comes to your mind, and how do you feel? Scared? Confident? Something else? Describe the image(s) and your feelings.

_____

_____

_____

_____

3. Now consider the five food boundaries against the various circumstances you encounter in day-to-day life. Pinpoint a specific area where you feel least confident in self-advocating for your life unbinged. Give yourself time for deep, inner exploration. Then write the circumstance, your feelings, and the whys and hows that shaped, or are currently influencing, your lack of confidence in advocating for your needs.

_____

_____

_____

_____

_____

4. Write about a specific circumstance when you didn't advocate for yourself. How did that play out? What was the end result? What were your feelings as you moved through the circumstance and afterward?

_____

_____

_____

_____

_____

_____

5. Write one or two statements you'd feel comfortable saying in such circumstances to advocate for yourself.

_____

_____

_____

_____

_____

_____

6. Which one of the following Scripture verses most keenly encourages your confidence to self-advocate for your life unbinged? Commit the verse to memory as a confidence booster:

☐ **Psalm 27:3**

Though an army besiege me [food], my heart will not fear [a life unbinged]; though war [temptation] break out against me, even then I will be confident [in self-advocating].

☐ **Joshua 1:9**

"Have I not commanded you? Be strong and courageous [living life unbinged]. Do not be afraid [to self-advocate]; do not be discouraged [about other people's feelings], for the Lord your God will be with you wherever you go."

☐ **Jeremiah 17:7**

Blessed is the one who trusts in the Lord, whose confidence is in him [each step of life unbinged, including self-advocating].

☐ **Philippians 1:6**

Being confident of this, that he who began a good work in you [life unbinged and self-advocating] will carry it on to completion until the day of Christ Jesus.

☐ **Hebrews 13:6**

"'The Lord is my helper; I will not be afraid [to self-advocate].'"

CHAPTER 18

Identifying the Enemy

The Enemy and Our Sinful Nature

JESUS CALLS SATAN THE FATHER OF LIES, THE DEVIL, AND THE THIEF WHO "COMES ONLY TO STEAL AND KILL AND DESTROY" (JOHN 10:10). Satan is the one behind all of our challenges and woes, taking advantage of our sin nature to trip us up and take us down.

The world calls him a saboteur or the oppressor, and many simply say "the universe" is out to get us. But don't be mistaken; Satan is real, alive, and in constant action against us. He's sly, strategic, and "prowls around like a roaring lion looking for someone to devour" (1 Peter 5:8)—anyone and everyone who's not paying attention, not watching, and not wearing the armor of God.

He's also sneaky. "Satan disguises himself as an angel of light" (2 Corinthians 11:14 ESV). Many times we don't recognize him. We go about our business, paying him no mind, often mistakenly thinking that what we're seeing is beautiful, so it must be good and from God. Why do we fall for the enemy's tricks? We haven't trained ourselves well to recognize him for what he truly is, which puts us right where he wants us: headed straight for a cliff. At times we don't even know the cliff or the ditch is in front of us because our enemy has disguised the road and decorated it with a whole lot of bling and sugar. In our day-to-day life, he's like the cruise ship activity director, hard at work to make sure the all-you-can-eat buffet is well-stocked and beautifully laid out and all of our sinful and unhealthy desires look too enticing to resist.

Like the cruise ship activity director, Satan's also an expert conversationalist and salesman, as we've seen from the beginning of time with Adam and Eve. He's the original expert at causing us to question what God has told us, and we end up making the grave error of leading others by the lies we've fallen for, just like Adam and Eve, who physically walked and talked with God. This is serious stuff.

Satan is adept at causing us to doubt and question and skew God's Word in favor of whatever we desire that appears and sounds good to us. He makes it easy for us to doubt God's love and question His best for us. Satan's wide road of hype is the dangerous road that leads to our destruction.

In the case of Eve, Satan told her that if God *really* loved her, He wouldn't withhold *anything* from her. The truth is this: While God our Father lavishes incredibly generous gifts and provision on us, He's also the Father who cautions us against, and sometimes withholds from us, what is not His best. Our part is to learn to distinguish between Satan's schemes and voice and God's work and voice by (1) studying and knowing the character of God, His instructions, and His cautions, and (2) knowing the character, lies, and disguises of the enemy.

When Satan's lies sound so logical (as they did to Adam and Eve), putting his spin on what God has said, we begin to doubt God. Whatever enticing thing we see before us that's not from God is Satan's work to make it appear *like* God and sound like Him. Why? Satan's mission is to get us to deny God and His Word and instead follow him. When we fall for Satan's lies in any way, big or small, we've moved ourselves outside of God's protective boundaries. Satan didn't move us; he just talked us into moving. Though believers in Jesus Christ cannot be snatched from God's hand (John 10:29), we can make choices that move us outside the perimeters of God's vast and beautiful garden of goodness that He created for joy, pleasure, fulfillment, health, and His glory, as He had the Garden of Eden.

God wants us to have great fun and fulfillment within the vast boundaries of His bountiful pleasures.

The Fall from Bounty

After God told Adam and Eve they could eat of *every* tree in the garden except the *one* in the middle, Satan came along and asked Eve, "Did God really say, 'You must not eat from any tree in the garden?'" (Genesis 3:1).

Eve replied about the single tree that was off limits: "God did say, 'You must not eat fruit from the tree that is in the middle of the garden . . . or you will die'" (Genesis 3:3).

Then Satan flat out lied. He said, "You will not certainly die" (Genesis 3:4), enticing them with the pride he'd shown in heaven when he said in his heart, "I will make myself like the Most High" (Isaiah 14:14).

An outright lie is sometimes easier to believe than a partial lie.

The enemy is the originator of lies with one agenda: to steal, kill, and destroy.

- He lies outright.
- He spins truth with partial lies.
- He totally dresses up what's harmful to make it look appealing.

No matter how his scheming sounds or how he's dressed it up, no matter how crafty and clever he is, no matter how seemingly "necessary" something he's offering seems, it is a lie.

Eve's Weaknesses and Mistakes

In Eve's encounter with Satan, the first thing she did was let her contentment be undermined by the enemy. All was great—perfect—in the garden stocked with superb food and heavenly ambiance. Yet when she looked at that one tree God said not to eat from, she became fixated on it, just as Satan had become fixated on being like God. And he brought that same appeal into the conversation, telling Eve, "You will be like God" (Genesis 3:5).

Aren't there times when we have this attitude: "I want what I want and I'm going to have it"? And once we get it, don't we, for a moment, feel like a goddess?

As was the case in the Garden of Eden, God has prepared for us countless amazing foods, colorful and delicious, for our enjoyment and health. Yet we allow Satan to undermine our contentment and God's goodness and protection over us.

Maybe I'm at a birthday party and someone says to me, "Don't be silly; you can have a piece of cake. What harm will *one* piece do? It's a birthday party. Live a little!" That kind of talk is like the persuasive voice of the enemy, causing me to question God's boundaries. If I'm not standing strong and rooted in the knowledge of God's best for me, I'm going to be swayed to think, *Maybe I am being silly and it's okay for me to eat just one piece. . . . Maybe I'm not as happy as I could be.*

> Blessed is the one who trusts in the Lord, whose confidence is in him. They will be like a tree planted by the water that sends out its roots by the stream. It does not fear when heat comes; its leaves are always green. It has no worries in a year of drought and never fails to bear fruit. (Jeremiah 17:7–8)

We can be moving along beautifully, bearing good fruit, and then we see or hear something so enticing or convincing that, all of a sudden, our happiness and contentment come into question. Are we rooted so deeply in Christ that we can't be that easily moved or not moved at all?

> Let your eyes look straight ahead; fix your gaze directly before you. Give careful thought to the paths for your feet and be steadfast in all your ways. Do not turn to the right or the left; keep your foot from evil. (Proverbs 4:25–27)

Eve was moved by temptation to think that God was withholding something potentially great from her, something more, something better, than the vast and effusive goodness He'd provided for her and Adam. Instead of stopping and checking her roots, she responded impulsively and took a bite. She hadn't even first talked with her husband, Adam, to gain his perspective on disobeying God. She handed the fruit to him, and he ate it too.

My guess is that she didn't first talk with Adam because she didn't want to take the chance of being talked out of eating the fruit. She "saw that the fruit of the tree was good for food and pleasing to the eye, and also desirable for gaining wisdom" (Genesis 3:6). She'd already made up her mind before she even thought about her accountability partner.

I've done the same thing.

At periods of time over the past years, I've desired a particular food, and had I reached out to someone who knew my food struggle—my husband, a friend, or one of my kids—I know they would have tried to talk me out of that self-harm I had oftentimes vowed to stand strong against. I don't always want to be talked out of what I want. How about you? I want to jump in, eat what I want, and keep my addiction hidden by not talking to anyone about it before or after. And the addiction grew bigger and bigger, like a monster eating me up.

As the father of lies, Satan gets a thrill out of us keeping secrets and living hidden in what's stealing, killing, and destroying us. Heck! We're taking some work off his hands—but we're adding to the weight of our hearts, minds, and bodies, as Eve and Adam discovered in the aftermath of their choice to sin against God.

God gave us each other not only for human companionship but also as a "suitable helper" (Genesis 2:21), for support, encouragement, and accountability.

> A cord of three strands is not quickly broken. (Ecclesiastes 4:12)

"Where two or three gather in my name, there am I with them."
(Matthew 18:20)

He began to send them out two by two and gave them authority over
impure spirits. (Mark 6:7)

When we're facing temptation, we need to call on God, revisit His Word, and call on others—our spouse, a friend, the person we can share honestly with—who will, in turn, be honest with us.

Kristy, don't give in to that! This is not what you really want. You can stand strong against this temptation.

Who are the trusted people in your life who will be frank with you and say no? After Eve jumped into sin, ate the forbidden fruit, and turned to Adam, he proved to be supportive of her disobedience to God by joining her in that sin.

It's easy to feel less guilty when somebody else is willing or eager to go along with giving in to temptation. We feel better about ourselves, in the moment, when we're with someone who is just as weak as we are. We need to surround ourselves with those who are strong in the Lord and strong in obedience, those who will truly have our backs by being honest.

Don't do that, Kristy! Run to God and worship Him.

Adam blamed Eve for his sin when God confronted him. And Eve blamed the serpent. Sound familiar? How many times has someone brought a special treat or meal that you knew was not inside your food boundaries? While eating is part of God's goodness to us, when we move outside of the boundaries of health because food has become our idol, that's sin. And what do we next do? We make excuses and blame others.

> Well, she brought that French vanilla latte to me as a gift, so I should drink it.

> It's my son's birthday, so I have to eat a piece of his cake.

> It's the office Christmas party; I don't want to be a prude.

> The church potluck is only once a month. So what's it going to hurt for me to have that roll and a brownie, just once?

We also lie to ourselves just as the enemy lies to us. There's never a "just once." Battling Satan is a daily, hourly, minute by minute, occasion by occasion, temptation by temptation choice. Why do we make it easier for him to steal, kill, and destroy us?

*We must take responsibility for our every
thought, choice, and action.*

Our choices are ours alone. We can't rightly blame anyone else for our actions. Yes, someone may make a surprise dessert for me, but if I choose to eat it when it's outside the boundary—not on the meal plan for the day or not food compliant—that's on me, the choice I made, my own responsibility.

Satan's Lies to You

What lies has the enemy told you? Have you heard these whispers in your mind?

- Just a little bite won't hurt. Just today. You can start again on Monday.
- You deserve this treat; you've been working so hard.
- Order that pizza, just this once.
- One bowl of ice cream won't hurt.
- Just one brownie.
- Just one little bag of chips.
- Do you really think God cares if you have just one? Of course not!

Lies.

Yes, God does care what I put in my body—this temple He fashioned for me to live in and glorify Him—and He gave me the responsibility to take the best care of this temple that I can.

I'm a person who always goes beyond "just one." God does care if I eat that bowl of ice cream because even with the best of intentions, I don't stop with one or two scoops.

We must learn to recognize Satan's voice and his lies, which are like "bindweed" he plants in our fertile minds. Bindweed got its name for a good reason:

> This fast-growing vine is one of the most aggressive, difficult perennial weeds to remove, and its little white morning-glory-like flowers [think of how Satan dresses traps to look so beautiful and enticing] produce lots of seeds. The main problem is with its white-rooted runners that spread deep and wide, making it very difficult to dig out. **Leave just a piece, and it will resprout.** These roots then become **mixed up with shrub and perennial roots and are hard to reach.** Moreover, **weed killers won't touch it.** Managing the weed in a three-step process is the only way to get rid of it.[9] (author emphasis)

We must be careful and watchful to avoid becoming *bound* by Satan's seeds of flowery lies. At the first whisper, "Just one bite. Just this time," we must take three steps to get rid of that root:

1. Take the thought captive to make it obedient to God—speaking truth to ourselves.
2. Take five deep breaths, pray, and praise, clothed in the armor of God.
3. Resist the devil by standing firm with your will surrendered to God's will.

It's in the stopping, praying, and walking away that we take captive our thoughts and surrender those bindweed seeds to God.

Once we begin to distinguish Satan's white morning glory lies from the truth, we will successfully overcome and do the next right thing.

We must practice distinguishing between falsehood and truth because Satan's mission in quickly multiplying lies is to steal, kill, and destroy us.

So what exactly does he want to steal from us, kill, and destroy?

- our confidence in Jesus Christ and His power, protection, provision, and great plans for us
- our strength and effectiveness to do the next right thing
- our joy, contentment, and love, and the boundaries that fortify and protect these
- our ability and effectiveness to take care of ourselves and minister to our kids, our spouses, and others
- our minds, discernment, and knowledge of truth
- our relationships and ability to engage in iron sharpening iron, encouraging others, and receiving encouragement

He wants us so bound up in his bindweed, producing and multiplying our sin, shame, and guilt, that we isolate ourselves from our Savior, our faith, our family, our health, our well-being, and the godly support of believers in Christ Jesus.

> ### *The enemy does his best work when we've bound ourselves in isolation.*

Once we're bound in isolation, Satan doesn't stop there. He continues to entice us with the deceivingly beautiful flowers that are actually vines of false hope, false freedom, false fixes. *Eat whatever you want, whenever you want; you're free to fill yourself!*

Those lies are what pulled me, bound me, and buried me in food addiction, just like the lies that pulled Eve and Adam into the bondage of sin.

We can't serve two masters.

When we're serving ourselves whatever we desire, whatever looks and feels good at any given time, we aren't serving our Father, nor are we living in the plentiful garden of His best that He created for our utmost fulfillment, enjoyment, and nourishment.

We're not just talking about food here; we're talking about our whole being: body, mind, spirit, relationships, finances, etc.

Once Satan has us bound, his intent is to keep us bound, naked, and ashamed, stripped of the armor of God and our righteousness (right living), stripped of all our defenses—the Word of God and His protection. The thing is, Satan didn't force us into those; we made our own decisions.

Consider this:

- When we're eating whatever we want—noncompliant foods—we're destroying our biological defenses against illness and disease.

- When we're feeding our minds whatever entices us—ungodly junk and the pain of our past—we're destroying our mental and emotional defenses, resulting in mental and emotional illnesses.

- When we're feeding on other people's ideas of spirituality instead of God's Word, or we're skewing His Word to fit our own agendas, we're destroying our spiritual defenses.

The breakdown or health of any of these areas (body, mind, and spirit) directly impacts the others. An unhealthy body adversely affects the mind and spirit. An unhealthy mind affects the body and spirit. An unhealthy spirit affects the mind and body.

By virtue of eating whatever we want, we're partnering with Satan in his intent to steal, kill, and destroy our body, mind, and spirit, which metastasizes to destroy our relationships and purposes and every other aspect of our lives. Satan wants us out of God's Word and turned away from truth because when we're feeding on God's Word, we're consistently reminded of His perfect plan, purpose, power, protection, and provision for us; His might, glory, and goodness for us; His cleansing and filling; and His fortification—His strength and power in us to make choices against the enemy and the things of this world he uses to harm and destroy us.

> Be on your guard; stand firm in the faith; be courageous; be strong.
> (1 Corinthians 16:13)

Action Step: Seeing and Feeling My Behavior—Part 1

What does it look and feel like when you're "in the food"? Draw that picture. Don't worry about your artistic skills; just get the idea of your behavior on paper.

Study what you've drawn and describe how the image and your thoughts make you feel.

_____

_____

_____

_____

_____

CHAPTER 19

Defeating the Enemy

Willing Spirit, Weak Flesh

MATTHEW 26:41 SAYS, "WATCH AND PRAY SO THAT YOU WILL NOT FALL INTO TEMPTATION. The spirit is willing, but the flesh is weak." Isn't that the truth!

How often do we sincerely want to make the next right decision but we don't? We fall face first into the ditch or over the cliff. We want to do the right thing, to honor God with our choices, but our flesh, our human nature, is weak when we choose to dismiss God's strength in us. We strengthen and fortify our "new self" (we are new creations in Christ Jesus by faith) by consistently feeding from the rich nutrients of God's Word and His Holy Spirit, who is ever at work in us. God does not stray from us; we stray from Him. God does not ban us from His banquet table; we don't accept His invitation to dine with Him.

> He satisfies the thirsty and fills the hungry with good things. (Psalm 107:9)

The best way to strengthen our nature as a new creation in Christ Jesus is to be in God's powerful, living Word every day: reading, studying, feasting on His Word at His table, and fellowshipping with Him through prayer.

I'll be honest with you. I don't wake up every day and think, *Yay! I can't wait to get into the Bible.* My first thought is often anything but the Bible: *I need to check my email, make breakfast for the kids, plan the curriculum for the day, and attend to whatever is going on.*

My instinct is not to run to God's table, though I know I need to be there first thing to ensure I'm fitted and fortified to keep doing the next right thing and well-equipped to extinguish every flaming arrow that Satan *will* shoot at me throughout the day.

He especially targets me in my kitchen and on the road, where he—the "angel of light"—has erected tall, bright fast-food signs with mouthwatering, larger-than-life pictures. He's everywhere we are and into everything we're doing. He's determined to trip us up and take us down whenever and wherever our defenses are weak.

Defeating the Enemy

God has given us everything we need to defeat the enemy every time.

- "Be alert and of sober mind" (1 Peter 5:8).
- "Reject every kind of evil" (1 Thessalonians 5:22).
- "Resist the devil, and he will flee from you" (James 4:7).
- "Do not give the devil a foothold" (Ephesians 4:27).
- "Test the spirits to see whether they are from God" (1 John 4:1).
- "Be strong in the Lord and in His mighty power" (Ephesians 6:10).
- "Put on the full armor of God, so that you can take your stand against the devil's schemes" (Ephesians 6:11).
- "Pray in the Spirit on all occasions with all kinds of prayers and requests. With this in mind, be alert and always keep on praying for all the Lord's people" (Ephesians 6:18).

The Armor of God

What is the armor God provides for us? What does it look like? What does putting on His armor actually mean in our day-to-day life? The apostle Paul introduced the armor of God and why we must stay fully fitted in the armor:

> Put on the **full armor** of God, so that you **can** take your stand against the devil's schemes. For our struggle is not against flesh and blood, but against the rulers, against the authorities, against the powers of this dark world and against the spiritual forces of evil in the heavenly realms. Therefore put on the **full armor** of God, so that **when** the day of evil comes, you may be **able** to stand your ground, and after you have done **everything, to stand. Stand firm then**, with the belt of **truth** buckled around your waist, with the breastplate of **righteousness** in place, and with your feet fitted with the **readiness** that comes from the gospel of peace. In addition to **all** this, take up the shield of **faith**,

with which you **can** extinguish **all** the flaming arrows of the evil one. Take the helmet of **salvation** and the sword of the Spirit, which is the **word of God**. (Ephesians 6:11–17, author emphasis)

Pay close attention to the bolded phrases and visit the additional Scripture verses:

- **full armor**—not just parts and pieces (Romans 13:12)

- **can**—we can "do all things through Christ who gives us strength" (Philippians 4:13)

- **when**—not if but when the day of evil (temptations) come (1 Corinthians 10:13)

- **able**—fully equipped and empowered to defeat the enemy (1 Corinthians 10:13)

- **everything, to stand**—applying all of God's instructions to be able to "stand firm then," and what remains is our *steel will* to stand, fully armored, no matter what (2 Peter 1:3–5)

- **truth**—(God's Word) who He says He is, who He says we are in Christ, truth about our addictions and fallibilities, truth about the enemy and God's redemption for us (John 17:17)

- **righteousness**—right living, taking the next right step no matter what (James 1:22–27)

- **readiness**—for temptations, for how Satan will next present himself to us, readiness to defeat Him with God's Word, readiness to give an answer for what we believe and why (1 Peter 3:15)

- **faith**—not in ourselves or others but full faith in the Lord Jesus Christ and God's living Word (Proverbs 3:5–6)

- **all**—extinguishing each and every fiery arrow Satan shoots at us (Colossians 1:10–11)

- **salvation**—faith and belief in Jesus Christ, faith that He has saved us forever and we cannot be snatched from our Father's hand, no matter what (John 10:29)

- **Word of God**—"alive and active, sharper than any double-edge sword" (Hebrews 4:12)

This is serious stuff! And not without reward. God often includes a promise when He gives instruction. Look back at Ephesians 6:11: "Put on the full armor of God, **so that you can take your stand** against the devil's schemes." He thereby assures us of the outcome every single time we obey Him.

Bonus Online Content

Recite the warriors prayer with Kristy.

Fight Through the Bite

Someone once shared this AA concept with me: think through the drink. Talking about that in one of my coaching groups, someone said, "Fight through the bite." I thought that twist was fantastic! Think fully through your food and craving situations, fighting through the bite, and see where that leads you. Let's say I'm at a party, potluck, restaurant, or drive-through and I want something that's not on my food plan. Here's what that spiraling inner *fight through the bite* challenge may sound like:

If I eat one bite of that, I'll have another bite.

Then what?

Well, I'll likely have a third bite and finish it off.

Then what?

I'm going to want more.

Then what?

I'm probably going to have more.

Then what?

I'm going to want more to binge on later.

Then what?

I'll want to sneak it out with me because people will have noticed that I've eaten too much already.

Then what?

I'll be filled with shame and guilt and anger.

Then what?

I'll go to sleep in that destroyed state, yet I'll repeat the cycle the next day because . . .

I've flung myself over the cliff and dug myself into a ditch.

The pause before the first bite, to think through all the truths, is powerful. Why? Because the truth can set us free from the ditch and cliff-diving of food addiction. Maybe you've heard this: One bite is too many and one thousand is never enough. True. That first bite is the first sprig of quickly multiplying vines of bindweed, distracting us by its beautiful white flowers. Before we know it, we've tripped on a vine and gotten ourselves bound up in it. Nobody ever wakes up wishing they had binged or overeaten the night before.

There are times when I walk into my pantry, preparing for dinner or putting something away, and Satan will whisper in my ear and point out the one thing that's not on the day's plan or a noncompliant food a family member stored there.

"Just eat one," he urges. That temptation food is what I call a "gateway" food. Matthew 7:13 says, "Wide is the gate and broad is the road that leads to destruction." There are certain foods, like salty nuts, that are plan-compliant but, for me, can be gateway foods that lead me straight into the addiction ditch. Even a compliant food eaten impulsively can lead to overeating. Sometimes I'll walk into the pantry and hear that call from the enemy, and I'll say out loud, "NO!" just as Jesus said, "Get thee behind me, Satan" (Matthew 16:23 KJV)!

My family often asks, "Who are you talking to?"

I'll tell them the truth. "Sometimes food calls to me. It's tempting, so I tell it no, loud and clear, and then I don't want it."

Perhaps talking to food seems weird, but I'll take that any time over falling prey to eating off-plan, obsessing over food, being overweight, and feeling trapped in the food bondage where I used to exist.

Instead of giving in to "just eat one," dig in and dig out that bindweed root with the firm spade of "NO!"

Willpower

We're all gifted with free will, but we don't always choose to use that power, at least not to its fullest. We may wake up in the morning with a strong mindset, ready to face the day, raring to go, feeling like we can conquer anything—until we hear Satan's whisper in the face of that noncompliant food.

I'd had a 5:00 a.m. meeting with a friend from my accountability group, and later that day I called her and said, "I'm really struggling, really tempted to eat a particular food. Will you pray for me? Can we walk through this?"

We did, and then she said, "You were so strong this morning at five o'clock."

"I'm always strong at five o'clock in the morning," I replied. "I can conquer the world at 5:00 a.m."

Give me until six, seven, or eight in the morning when I'm in the throes of life—doctors' appointments, housecleaning, laundry, phone calls, etc.—and my willpower is depleting. If I don't pause throughout the day to recharge, I'll hit the ditch and fling my food plan over the cliff by making choices I don't want to make. Here's a visual:

Let's say we're in a video game, like Super Mario Bros., and we're losing power. The way to rebuild power is to gather gold coins, which is great, except in real life. Can we gather gold coins while running errands and taking care of the house, kids, pets, and friends? No. When our internal power bar drops like Super Mario Bros.' power meter, here are some gold coins that recharge us to do the next right thing:

- reading and reciting God's Word
- getting on our knees and saying, "Lord, I need help this afternoon! Recharge me!"
- having a one-minute dance party to a worship or praise song
- calling a friend and asking her to pray for us

What time of day is particularly hard for you? For me, it's 3:00 p.m. hands down, every afternoon. When I have a tempting thought, I'll sometimes grab a sparkling water and call a friend who understands my struggle. I set an alarm on my phone for 3:00 p.m. to remind me to pause, and I get away from the bustle and stress by taking a few minutes to recharge my willpower back to 100 percent.

There are times when we're white-knuckling our way through the day. Perhaps you have an event to attend and you're repeating to yourself, *I'm not going to eat. I'm not going to eat. I'm not going to eat.* You're gritting your teeth to get through the day and the event. But white-knuckling and teeth-gritting aren't always successful. Seeking the treasures of God is.

We must pause, breathe, pray, and praise to recharge our willpower.

Each of the pause steps I've shared in this book is a powerful gold coin you can pick up throughout your day:

- the gold coin of prayer
- the gold coin of worship
- the gold coins in the Word of God (a treasure trove)
- the gold coin of connecting with an accountability friend

Action Step: Seeing and Feeling My Behavior—Part 2

What does it look like when you're *not* "in the food" and you're fully surrendered to God's best?

Study what you've drawn and describe how the image and your thoughts make you feel.

_____

_____

_____

_____

_____

CHAPTER 20

The Holy Spirit and His Work in Us

Who Is the Holy Spirit?

THE HOLY SPIRIT IS ONE PERSON OF THE TRIUNE GODHEAD—FATHER, SON, AND SPIRIT—CO-EQUAL AND CO-ETERNAL. I love Billy Graham's explanation of God's Spirit: "Today the Holy Spirit illuminates the minds of people, makes us yearn for God, and takes spiritual truth and makes it understandable to us."[10]

When we accept Jesus as our Savior, God's Spirit enters us and then permanently dwells in us as our supreme guide, counselor, comforter, power, strength, encourager, intercessor, protector, and teacher, who is ever-present in us, no matter what.

That phrase "no matter what" will be important for you to keep in mind as we delve deeply into the topic of grieving the Holy Spirit and the natural consequences of that choice, and also the choice to bring joy to God.

The Holy Spirit Intercedes for Us

Jesus said,

"If you love me, you will keep my commandments. And I will ask the Father, and he will give you another Helper, to be with you forever, even the Spirit of truth, whom the world cannot receive, because it neither sees him nor knows him. You know him, for he dwells with you and will be in you." (John 14:15–17 ESV)

When we pray to God our Father, His Holy Spirit intercedes on our behalf. He helps us navigate this hard life and every challenge we face.

We don't always know what we're feeling, so we don't always know what to pray. But the Holy Spirit knows. He knows our every thought, feeling, need, and desire, and He speaks to the Father on our behalf when we don't know how or what to share with Him. The Spirit of God is our comforter when we just need to cry out in our desperation, frustration, grief, and pain but have no words. He intervenes with comfort and speaks to the Father what we cannot utter or coherently express.

> The Spirit helps us in our weakness. We do not know what we ought to pray for, but the Spirit himself intercedes for us through wordless groans. (Romans 8:26)

The Spirit also shows us the way as our counselor and guide. He empowers us to be able to make it through circumstances we otherwise, on our own, could not manage.

No matter your state of mind, when you want to talk to God but don't know what to say or how to convey your thoughts and feelings because they're too mixed up inside you, God hears you clearly through His Spirit in you. He simply wants us to come to Him even when we can't put two words together. He is always in us, interceding for us, comforting us, guiding us—a beautiful part of our intimate, divine relationship with our Creator.

Consider how very much God loves you that He would gift such a powerful part of Himself to reside in you to keep you connected to Him, no matter what, even when you don't know what to say or think or how you feel. God does, all the time, in every moment, because His Spirit is living in you, is at work in and through you, and is interceding for you in every way. This includes giving you everything you lack—strength, knowledge, understanding, guidance, and comfort—sharing in your heartaches and joy, and more. In other words, we are made whole by the Spirit of God at work in us.

The Holy Spirit Teaches Us

John 14:26 assures us that "the Helper, the Holy Spirit, whom the Father will send in my name, he will teach you all things and bring to your remembrance all that I have said to you" (ESV). How incredible is this as well! Oh, the power within us!

When did I last thank and praise God for His Spirit within me?

The Holy Spirit gives us insight and clarity when we're reading the Bible and biblically sound devotions, when we're listening to biblically sound sermons and teachings, when we're praying and worshipping, and even when we're talking with others about the Word. When we read or hear something that's inconsistent or otherwise inaccurate according to His Word, it's the Holy Spirit in us who gives us pause, brings truth to our minds, and prompts us to go straight to the Word for truth.

When we're going through something—anything—and a Scripture verse, a comforting thought, an answer, or clarity comes to mind, that's the work of the Holy Spirit teaching us and reminding us that our help is always near, always present. When we're in a time when we need God's Word and guidance (which is all the time), He brings to mind exactly what we need to hear.

When did you last attribute to the Holy Spirit an internal "knowing" or a Scripture verse that came to mind?

Our part is in spending time studying His Word. God's Spirit works in tandem with us— with the brain He gave us to read, reason, memorize, and engage in critical thinking. If we're memorizing Scripture, we are rewarded with remembrance of the verses or passages when we need them.

When we're faithful to read God's Word, He will also use us to share His Word from memory with others in their time of need. Have you ever experienced a time when you were talking with a friend and a Scripture verse that was fitting for your friend's circumstance popped into your mind? That's the very present work of the Holy Spirit through you because you're doing your part to store God's Word in your heart (Psalm 119:11). Such times are not to bring us glory, but to help care for others in their time of need and to draw them to read and learn God's Word for themselves. And thus, the gospel multiplies and spreads.

The Holy Spirit also tunes our thoughts to the voice of the Father. There are times when God's Spirit will call on us to do difficult, challenging, uncomfortable work, which is why it's extremely important that we learn to *clearly* differentiate between (1) the voice of the Holy Spirit, (2) the enemy's voice, (3) our own voice, and (4) the voice of parents, teachers, and others whose voices are embedded in us.

We can learn to recognize God's voice, remembering we are always "yoked" with Christ and have a responsibility to listen in order to learn to distinguish His voice from other voices by consistently reading, studying, and memorizing His Word to be a "worker . . . who correctly handles the word of truth" (2 Timothy 2:15).

Know that the Holy Spirit's voice will *never* contradict His written Word because they are one and the same. "The Word was with God, and the Word was God" (John 1:1).

When God calls us to do something challenging, at times our own voices will say, *Oh, no! Not me! I'm can't do that; it's too hard. I'm not skilled in that. I'm too shy to talk to that person about that.* But the Holy Spirit empowers us and helps us to be in tune with His voice by bringing to our remembrance His Word, His teaching, and how He's been shaping and empowering us to be all God created us to be for His purpose and glory—"for such a time as this" (Esther 4:14).

How blessed we are! We are chosen. We have the very Spirit of God at work in and through us.

The Holy Spirit Gives Us Peace, Hope, and Love

Romans 5:1–3 is a beautiful passage that affirms we have in us God's peace, hope, love, and rejoicing—no matter what:

> Since we have been made right in God's sight by faith, we have **peace** with God because of what Jesus Christ our Lord has done for us. Because of our faith, Christ has brought us into this place of undeserved privilege where we now stand, and we confidently and joyfully look forward to sharing God's glory.
>
> We can **rejoice**, too, when we run into problems and trials, for we know that they help us develop endurance. And endurance develops strength of character, and character strengthens our **confident hope** of salvation. And this hope will not lead to disappointment. For we **know** how dearly **God loves us**, because he has given us the Holy Spirit to fill our hearts with his **love**. (author emphasis)

We can rejoice in our suffering? Yes! Why? Because God is always at work for our good and even produces good from our suffering. How?

- Endurance and perseverance develop our
- strength of character, which in turn strengthens our
- confident hope, which cannot disappoint. Why?
- Because we "know how dearly God loves us." How do we know?
- He gave us His Holy Spirit to "fill our hearts with His love."

Do you see that never-ending circle of God's faithfulness? Even if we can't *feel* God's love at times, we can be confident that we are *filled* with His love through the Holy Spirit in us. Knowing this truth becomes more and more evident as we push through our challenges with endurance and willpower, staying yoked with Christ and doing the next right thing.

We may not *feel* God's love when we're battling against the buffet, but with the conscious and confident knowledge that we are *filled* with God's Spirit and His love and power, we can endure to the other side through each next right step. What is the work of God's love in us?

> Love bears all things [regardless of what comes], believes all things [looking for the best in each one], hopes all things [remaining steadfast during difficult times], endures all things [without weakening]. (1 Corinthians 13:7 AMP)

Wow! That verse is important to memorize and apply in every circumstance. As we endure trials, the Holy Spirit helps us remember God's love—a love beyond our ability to understand.

We can apply the apostle Paul's prayers over us. These are also important verses to memorize:

> I pray that you, being rooted and established in love, may have power, together with all the Lord's holy people, to grasp how wide and long and high and deep is the love of Christ, and to know this love that surpasses knowledge—that you may be filled to the measure of all the fullness of God. (Ephesians 3:17–19)

> May the God of hope fill you with all joy and peace as you trust in Him, so that you may overflow with hope by the power of the Holy Spirit. (Romans 15:13)

The power of the Holy Spirit allows us to have, experience, and know God's peace, power, confidence, courage, hope, and extraordinary love in ways we could never attain on our own. God is so good and faithful to us!

The Holy Spirit Is Our Guide

What thoughts and feelings does the term *guide* stir in you?

The Holy Spirit "will guide you into all the truth" (John 16:13).

That verse doesn't say God forces us into all truth, right? He guides with "a gentle whisper" (1 Kings 19:12) and grace (Hebrew 10:29).

Since we are "yoked" with Christ, the Spirit in us, what is our part? Our work? A good picture of this is a child who's being guided by a parent through the child's bedtime routine. There are times when that routine isn't a smooth passage. Why?

*To be guided by the Holy Spirit, we must be willing,
listening, following, and surrendering.*

When we're willing, listening, following, and surrendering to the Holy Spirit's whisper in us, we'll be gently guided into all truth. The Spirit guides us with love, gentleness, and patience. Remember this as we move deeper.

When a voice is screaming inside you—*You really messed up! You're hopeless!*—you can be certain that the voice is not the Holy Spirit's. Paying attention to our thoughts, taking every thought captive, we begin to distinguish who is speaking in us.

- **The Holy Spirit's voice** is always gentle and loving as He reminds us of truth, guides us, teaches us, and corrects us.

- **Our own voices and the voices from our relationships** vacillate between pressure and praise, condemnation and encouragement, and screaming and whispering. In other words, they are unstable and not firmly reliable.

- **Satan's voice** is always lying, no matter what, and always contradictory to God's Word. His voice vacillates. Sometimes he whispers beautiful words. At other times, his words are dreadful, hideous, confusing, and mocking. Either way, they are never reliable.

Returning to the scenario of guiding a child through their bedtime routine, God the Father is faithfully patient, loving, gentle, and kind in guiding us. And we (His children) are often willful, not always cooperative, submissive, or obedient under His care.

As we practice surrendering our every thought and will to obey Christ, we grow spiritually mature. Our lives become far more peaceful, calm, fun, adventurous, fulfilling, and safe. We become ready to disciple others. But to arrive at that level of spiritual maturity, we must practice, just as children practice as they grow up.

- **Practice listening** for His voice and to His voice. He chooses from a number of ways to speak to us:
  - during our prayers
  - while we're reading His Word
  - in the Scripture verses we've memorized
  - in the promptings we receive from the Holy Spirit
  - through others

- **Practice hearing** Him and learning to distinguish His voice from human voices and Satan's well-groomed voice.
- **Practice surrendering**, trusting, and obeying God's voice in faith.

We can certainly feel lost when any of those three practices are not in play. Growing in them requires intentionality. When we've learned to recognize the Holy Spirit's voice and we've surrendered to His leadership, we don't feel lost, confused, fearful, directionless, helpless, or hopeless because He always—always—leads us into truth. We can then act on the truth with *confidence*, wherein comes peace, contentment, and joy, which is the strength of the Lord at work in us.

How often do we choose our spouse, a friend, a pastor, a counselor, a book, a sermon, and Google search for answers and guidance, excluding the Holy Spirit? It's not that those earthly sources are bad. God's Word tells us to seek and listen to wise counsel (Proverbs 19:20; 20:18). The issue is who is *leading*. Is it a human, Satan, or the Holy Spirit of God and His Word?

Plenty of times, I needed an answer and went straight to Google, bypassing any thought of the Holy Spirit and His Word. Or I'd go to my husband or ask my friends what I should do. Again, God may very well use human sources, but I should "seek *first* the kingdom of God and his righteousness" (Matthew 6:33 ESV, author emphasis).

God the Father is the One with all the answers and all truth. His Spirit will sometimes lead us to a human source for further understanding, reminders, teaching, correction, and affirmation. Then the question is this: Does the information align with God's Word? That reminds us of the importance of reading, studying, and memorizing the Word under the teaching of the Holy Spirit. He alone is the One who ensures and assures us we're on the right path, His path, the narrow path through the narrow gate.

Action Step: Learn to Recognize God's Voice

Consider your recent thoughts. Write those thoughts and identify the true voice: (1) your voice, (2) another human's voice, (3) the enemy's voice, or (4) the Holy Spirit's voice.

Recent Thought(s)	True Voice
_____	_____
_____	_____
_____	_____
_____	_____
_____	_____
_____	_____
_____	_____
_____	_____
_____	_____

CHAPTER 21

Let Us Not Grieve
the Holy Spirit

What does it mean to *grieve* the Holy Spirit?

ANYTHING UNACCEPTABLE TO GOD IS A SOURCE OF GRIEF TO THE HOLY SPIRIT. If you have children, you've had times of grief when they went against your wise counsel or directive. You were grieved because you love them with every fiber of your being and want only the very best for them.

Now imagine God's love for you, His child, a love far greater than the enormous love you have for others. Sit with that truth. It's mind-boggling, so great a love that it's beyond our ability to comprehend.

Consider the word "filling," which relates to our stomachs, our spirits, and the Holy Spirit.

- How often have you heard about "the filling of the Holy Spirit"?
- How often do you think about "filling" yourself?

Combining those two thoughts, let's looks at Ephesians 5:18 as an example. "Do not get drunk on wine, which leads to debauchery. Instead, be *filled* with the Spirit" (author emphasis). Other versions of the Bible translate *debauchery* as "wild living" (ISV), "excess" (KJV), "reckless" (BSB). Merriam-Webster's definition is "extreme indulgence in bodily pleasures."[11]

What is your extreme indulgence in bodily pleasures?

Mine was overeating and bingeing. I wanted to feed myself indulgently for the temporary feel-good filling and feeling. Our self-indulgences are never lasting and those indulgences grieve the Holy Spirit. In your efforts to fill yourself, have you noticed how fleeting the feel-good feeling is? Yet I wanted what I wanted, addicted to that temporary "hit" of sugary sweets. My food pursuits were all about me, me, me rather than God's best, His will, for me. I was (and am) completely selfish in so many areas, and food is my greatest struggle.

His best is that I surrender my will and ways to His because His are *the* best. He's our good, good Father who only gives the best of the best. His best never runs empty, always satisfies, and strengthens us in every way—body, mind, emotions, and spirit.

> The Lord will *always* lead you, satisfy you in a parched land, and strengthen your bones. You will be like a watered garden and like a spring whose water never runs dry. (Isaiah 58:11 CSB, author emphasis)

Overeating (gluttony) is extreme, self-serving, and greedy. Gluttony results in recklessness (lack of self-control) to the point of sickness, bloating, all-over pain, and excess weight. It causes our physical heart to work harder and our blood pressure to rise, inviting diabetes and other illnesses and diseases, including mental illnesses. Any greed and recklessness certainly grieves the Holy Spirit and has natural consequences.

> Drunkards and gluttons become poor, and drowsiness clothes them in rags. (Proverbs 23:21)

These behaviors pull us away from God, His purpose, and what is best for us. They embody lowering His supremacy (authority and rule over all things as Creator) and raising self, selfishness, pride, greed, recklessness, disorder, laziness, etc., as higher than Him. Anything we place as more important than God, as portrayed by our attitudes and actions, is sin and associated with idolatry and greed.

Recall your worst food phase. Maybe it was recent or years ago. Would you consider that reckless? Would you consider that God-honoring?

> "I have the right to do anything," you say—but not everything is beneficial. (1 Corinthians 6:12)

> Sodom's sins were pride, gluttony, and laziness, while the poor and needy suffered outside her door. (Ezekiel 16:49 NLT)

> Their god is their appetite, they brag about shameful things, and they think only about this life here on earth. (Philippians 3:19 NLT)

We grieve the Holy Spirit when leading our lives by the desires of our flesh (greed), doing whatever we want, whenever we want, which is the "wide gate" and "broad road that leads to destruction" (Matthew 7:13).

When serving ourselves food with reckless abandon and greed,

- **our bodies** become like a wide gate and broad road,
- **our minds and emotions** become like a wide gate and broad road, leaving us feeling lost and confused and searching, and
- **our spirits** become like a wide gate and broad road, a dry desert of dry bones, void of peace, joy, and contentment.

Let's be clear: Eating ice cream or fast food is not a *sin*. Overeating is.

For me, and possibly you, to dip into a bowl of ice cream or visit a drive-through is a wide gate with neon signs inviting me to wide and broad indulgence. In other words, lack of self-control. Eating a cupcake is not a sin if the intent and actual outcome is eating *one*. When we indulge in multiple cupcakes, we enter the wide gate.

For example, when I choose to eat a cupcake or bag of chips, my indulgence doesn't stop. I'm traveling down the wide road of my destruction. My *overindulgence* and food addiction grieve the Holy Spirit because I've diverted from His best for me—the plenty within boundaries. In those moments of temptation—before I even pick up my food nemesis—the Holy Spirit is whispering to me (trying to get my attention), wanting me to turn to Him, hear Him, see His best for me, and surrender to His best instead of my addiction. He wants me to cry out to Him for help the moment I see the wide gate.

We know our flesh (our will) is weak and a mess. We know what it feels like to be in a struggle without help. We lose the powerful help of the Holy Spirit when we turn to our own ways. But God promises a better way:

> ### *We are never alone in our struggles! God always makes a way of escape from entering the wide gate.*

> God is faithful. He will not allow the temptation to be more than you can stand. When you are tempted, he will show you a way out so that you can endure. (1 Corinthians 10:13)

The Holy Spirit will not force us into righteousness (right living) because He wants us to *choose Him*. So when I choose to ignore Him and His Word, I'm grieving Him.

Pride Grieves the Holy Spirit

When we're prideful, thinking, *I got this; I can do this on my own, in my own way,* and we're white-knuckling our way through a situation, what we're actually saying to the Holy Spirit is, "I don't need You, God, and I don't need the power of Your Spirit."

Confidence birthed by pride comes straight from our enemy. Yet we allow pride to be a barrier across the narrow gate and road that is God's best for us. "Narrow" is subjective and means within the boundaries of God's plenty, as with the vast Garden of Eden.

Pride prompts us to enter the wide gate, and a haughty spirit is a pothole along the wide road, causing us to fall needlessly and hurt ourselves, which hurts God because He's our Father.

> Pride goes before destruction, a haughty spirit before a fall. (Proverbs 16:18)

To turn from Satan's prompts, to avoid the wide ride and the falls, we must intentionally surrender ourselves, our ways, our desires, our pride, and our greed to God. We must remain within His boundaries, open to Him, and fully surrendered to Him. With that determined mindset, we experience the great work of the Holy Spirit in us:

Transformation!

Intentionality

Frankly, the last thing I want to do is grieve the Holy Spirit or restrain His power available to me. I'm sure you feel the same. I desire to live righteously, filled with the Holy Spirit. Thereby, we must be intentional with every choice.

> Intention: "a determination to act in a certain way."[12]

Intentionality is a powerful ingredient for righteous living:

1. Intentionally learn what behaviors grieve and restrain the Holy Spirit.
2. Intentionally practice these safeguards:

   - pausing
   - wearing every piece of God's armor
   - fleeing from Satan—stepping away or driving away from the temptation
   - taking God's way of escape
   - breathing
   - praying
   - weighing your choices against the natural consequences

- worshipping
- reading or reciting the Word
- calling an accountability friend

The Holy Spirit's Interceding

Think of the times you considered doing something you shouldn't, whether food-related or not. You had a sense, a nudge in your spirit that said, *I probably shouldn't do this.* That nudge was from the Holy Spirit, reminding you of the hazards of moving outside the boundaries and onto the wide road.

Maybe you were heading toward a drive-through while Satan was painting enticing pictures of fast food in your mind. The Holy Spirit interceded through a red traffic light, giving you a moment to consider your choices. Or He lowered the arms of a railroad crossing as you approached the track, giving you a lengthier pause to ponder the next right thing.

Have you considered that such instances are the Holy Spirit at work in you, giving you extra time to compare the consequences of your way with His best?

God is gracious; He doesn't force us into a decision, but such incidences of forced pause can be viewed as the interceding work of the Holy Spirit because 1 Corinthians 10:13 says, "When you are tempted, he will also provide a way out." That verse indicates that He's taking action to help you as He promised—not to make the decision for you but to give you extra time to stop and think instead of traveling at full speed over the cliff.

The decision to take His way out is on you. The Holy Spirit will tug at your heart to take the next right step, to stay in the safety of the boundaries, but it's your responsibility to "tune your ears to wisdom, and concentrate on understanding" (Proverbs 2:2). Surrendering to His best saves you from self-destruction.

Natural Consequences of Grieving the Holy Spirit

We must remember throughout this section that the sins of believers in Jesus Christ are covered, once and for all, by His blood—our past sins, present sins, and future sins—and nothing, not even our sin nature, can snatch us from Him (John 10:10).

We humans, bearing a sin nature, will continue to make mistakes and willful choices. It's our willfulness that drives us into the addiction ditch or over the cliff. Whether innocent mistakes or willful sin, both result in *natural consequences*, just as surrendering to God, obeying Him, and staying within healthy boundaries result in natural consequences.

Though God's grace, love, forgiveness, presence, and other gifts don't change, and He doesn't take them from us, there are still consequences. "If we go on sinning *deliberately* after receiving the knowledge of the truth, there no longer remains a sacrifice for sins" (Hebrews 10:26 ESV, author emphasis). In other words, when we *deliberately* sin, we are discounting God's goodness toward us and also the great sacrifice Christ made on our behalf.

Those facts should give us great pause.

The apostle Paul wrote about believers continuing to *choose* sin. He asked (rhetorically), "Should we keep on sinning so that God can show us more and more of his wonderful grace? Of course not! . . . Do not let sin *control* the way you live; do not *give in to* sinful desires. Do not let any part of your body become an instrument of evil to serve sin" (Romans 6:1–2, 12–13 NLT, author emphasis).

He's talking about exercising self-control and fully surrendering ourselves to the Holy Spirit.

> Instead, *give yourselves completely to God* [a choice, a decision, an action of our will], for you were dead, but now you have *new life*. So *use your whole body* as an instrument to *do what is right for the glory of God. Sin is no longer your master*, for you no longer live under the requirements of the law. Instead, you live under the freedom of God's grace. (Romans 6:13–14 NLT, author emphasis and explanations)

In other words, the choice to strengthen your self-control by the power of the Holy Spirit at work in you is your choice to make. Though you are forgiven, you still have the choice to sin or to exercise self-control—just as was the case for Adam and Eve.

Watch this domino effect of sin (the natural consequences):

When we choose to sin, Satan uses guilt and shame to trigger in us the sense that God no longer loves us and we can forget the many Bible verses that speak of His unfailing, faithful love.

Those barriers (guilt and shame) **block our confidence** in the truth of His abiding love. Think of it like this: What are your thoughts after you willfully sin? Likely, you think, *God can't possibly love me now or as much because I've sinned against Him.* Such thoughts are traps set by the father of lies, Satan.

Then we depart from the boundaries set by God for our utmost well-being, fulfillment, joy, and peace, and enter Satan's territory. Think of it like this: You walk beyond the perimeters of your home, into the woods, the hunters' zone, where you step on a camouflaged trap. Likewise, Satan's traps injure us, wreaking havoc on our minds, emotions, and lives.

> **We lose our sense of God's presence with us**, even though God said, "I will never leave you nor forsake you" (Hebrews 13:5 ESV). When we choose to sin, we move into hiding, blocking our awareness of His ever-presence, which is exactly how Adam and Eve felt in hiding.

As a child, when I did something my parents told me not to do, I'd run and hide in guilt and shame. We may try to hide from God, but He always finds us.

> Where can I go from your Spirit?
>   Where can I flee from your presence?
> If I go up to the heavens, you are there;
>   if I make my bed in the depths, you are there.
> If I rise on the wings of the dawn,
>   if I settle on the far side of the sea,
> even there your hand will guide me,
>   your right hand will hold me fast.
> If I say, "Surely the darkness will hide me
>   and the light become night around me,"
> even the darkness will not be dark to you;
>   the night will shine like the day,
>   for darkness is as light to you.

> (Psalm 139:7–12)

Just as God sought out Adam and Eve, He looks for us, calls us by name, uncovers our hiding place, searches our hearts, and corrects us. Why? Because He's our loving Father who wants us to know His love and presence (no matter what) and learn the importance of His boundaries that ensure our safety and protection from self-destruction.

Again, His grace is not a *license* for us to sin but a *learning* through sin's natural consequences:

> **Hiding after sinning, we lose the joy and strength of our salvation.** Nehemiah 8:10 says, "The joy of the Lord [fellowship with God] is your strength." God doesn't remove His joy and strength from us; we've chosen to move away from those gifts into enemy territory, where it's terrifying.

Are you happy in Christ, joyful in praise, worship, and life when you've willfully sinned? I'm certainly not. When you're without joy, do you feel strong? I don't. I feel strongest when I'm in right relationship with God—with no barriers between us.

We lose our sense of purpose, magnified by the devil's lies: *See, you're no good. You can't do anything right. You're not worthy of a purpose because you keep messing it up.* In enemy territory, you've chosen to leave your purpose behind. But God, the good shepherd who leaves the ninety-nine to find the one lost sheep and then rejoices (Matthew 18:10–14), never loses sight of His purpose for you. His Word says, "He who began a good work in you will carry it on to completion until the day of Christ Jesus" (Philippians 1:6), the day you meet Christ face to face.

Then we lose our sense of abundance, peace, calm—the joy factors.

Part of the Holy Spirit's abundance is the cornucopia of our experiences with Him— the times of His embrace, when He folds us in His arms of love, sings over us, nurtures us, and reminds us that we belong to Him and always will and that we're His heirs, His daughters, His princesses.

His faithful attention and love result in our peace and calm. When we choose to sin, moving into enemy territory—a dark, dense wood of camouflage—we can no longer see God's abundance. We're buried in abundant natural consequences, reaping fears and anxieties.

Choosing to live in enemy territory, we've left behind all the goodness and fortification of God's boundaries, including the armor of God. We are snared, naked, and terrified in enemy territory. Have you been there? Have you experienced the domino effect of natural consequences? Where do you usually end up? Trapped in the dark, dense wood of food addiction.

> *A beauty of the Holy Spirit of God is that we can return to Him with humble repentance and ask Him to rekindle His work in our hearts and lives.*

He is a good, good Father.

Fill Your Cup

How do you refill when your mind, body, or spirit feels depleted, as though your strength and willpower have diminished or vanished? My habit was to refill with sodas, sugary lattes, and noncompliant or unplanned food.

In such times, we can, instead, "approach God's throne of grace with confidence, so that we may receive mercy and find grace to help us in our time of need" (Hebrews 4:16).

Give deep thought to these poetic truths: The Holy Spirit "is able to do exceedingly abundantly *above all that we ask or think*, according to the power that works in us" (Ephesians 3:20 NKJV, author emphasis). An aspect of the Holy Spirit's work is to fill us to overflowing with the abundance of His kingdom. He invites us to His banquet table and invites us to ask for what we need and desire, whether daily, hourly, or minute by minute. He said that when we ask, we will receive, according to His will. As the greatest Father, He provides—in abundance—all that is *best* for us, and His abundance is enjoyable.

The apostle Paul prayed over us, "May the God of hope fill you with all joy and peace as you trust in him, so that you may overflow with hope by the power of the Holy Spirit" (Romans 15:13).

But what is our part? Our work with Him?

Imagine your water bottle has run dry. You're thirsty and need a refill. If you sit there, looking at the empty bottle, you'll become dehydrated. It's not the thought of refilling the bottle that makes the difference; it's your actions: engaging your willpower, getting up and taking the bottle to the water source, opening the bottle, allowing the source to fill it, and then drinking from it.

That's the picture of us "yoked together" with the Holy Spirit's work in us. He is the source of living water. We must carry our needs and desires to the fountain of God; open ourselves at His feet in prayer; by reading His Word, open our hearts and allow Him to fill us, knowing He is God, Jehovah Jireh (our Provider); and continue to consume His living water.

Fill me, Lord.

He will fill us. But will we set His provisions aside in favor of something else?

Action Step: My Letter to Food

Pause and ponder your relationship with food, then write a letter to food, considering these questions:

- How has your relationship with food harmed you over the years?
- Has the relationship trapped you?
- What has your relationship with food taken away from you?
- What other negative aspects of that relationship have impacted your life? Think deep and wide. How has it impacted your physical health and abilities, your emotional and mental health, and your relationships with people and with God?
- How do you want your relationship with food to look moving forward?

Dear Food,

_____

_____

_____

_____

_____

_____

_____

_____

PART 4

True Freedom

CHAPTER 22

Facing Your Feelings

FEELINGS CAN BE SO BIG AND SCARY AT TIMES THAT WE'D RATHER STUFF THEM DOWN BY ANY MEANS, LIKE BINGEING, THAN BE ALONE WITH THEM IN HEALTHY PROCESSING. Feelings are part of our nature and God's. We just don't often do so well when our feelings feel bigger than we think we can endure.

When Jesus walked the earth, He showed His feelings. At times He was sad. Other times He was angry. When He asked God to take the crucifixion "cup" from Him (Luke 22:42), I think He may have been experiencing what we know as desperation and fear of the physical torture He was facing. What an enormous sacrifice Christ made on our behalf so we wouldn't have to endure the consequences of our sins against our holy God!

When Christ ascended into heaven after His resurrection, He gifted us with the Holy Spirit to help us face and navigate our most difficult feelings with courage. Rather than stuff our feelings, He created us to feel them, as He does. He even gave us a multitude of Scriptures with promises that point to specific difficult feelings to remind us of these truths:

- God is always with us—always. We are never alone with our feelings (Matthew 28:20).

- "God is our refuge and strength, an ever-present help in trouble" (Psalm 46:1).

- When yoked with God, all things are possible—even facing our feelings (Matthew 19:26).

- God is our infinite source of divine peace, so much so that His peace (when we turn to Him) surpasses our human understanding (Philippians 4:7).

No word from God will ever fail.

(Luke 1:37)

Feelings are never wrong, but what we choose to do with them can be. Many people falsely believe that anger is a sin. The truth is that sin can result from what we choose to do with our anger. For example, it's not wrong to feel angry when someone hurts us. However, we move into sin when we let that anger fester and boil over into our words and actions, causing us, in turn, to hurt others.

Ignoring our feelings doesn't work either. Imagine a rubber ball in a sink full of water. What happens when you force the ball down? It pops back up to the surface. That's an example of trying to stuff down our feelings. The bigger the feelings, the bigger the ball, and regardless of size, that ball of feelings will resurface after we stuff it down.

Instead, we can face our feelings with God. His Word instructs us: "*In every situation, . . . present your requests to God*" (Philippians 4:6, author emphasis). Jesus said, "Come to me, all you who are weary and burdened, and I will give you rest" (Matthew 11:28).

Those Scripture verses are among many that tell us to face our feelings with God.

Feeling your feelings is the starting place to gain true healing and inner freedom.

The most healing way to release dark feelings is to open your heart and mind to God with honesty and thanksgiving. Why does our Father tell us to give thanks in all circumstances (1 Thessalonians 5:18)—thereby in all feelings? Perhaps because "in all things God works for the good of those who love him" (Romans 8:28).

While writing this book, a friend called me and shared that she was struggling hard. I could tell she needed to feel her feelings. She needed to sit with herself quietly and cry as she searched her heart to understand all that she was feeling and why. It would be a process. I encouraged her, "You need a big, ugly cry—a big, long, ugly cry."

"I don't have time for a big, long, ugly cry," she answered.

I countered honestly, thinking of how often I had felt as she was feeling. "Do you have time *not to* have that big, long, ugly cry?"

She replied honestly, "I'm afraid if I start crying, I won't stop."

I understood that feeling too. Sometimes, we start crying and don't stop because there's a forceful river of yucky feelings we've stored up behind a dam. Isn't that tremendous pressure how we sometimes feel? But we often push down hard on that big ball. Once the valve is surrendered, the tears are freed to begin their healing work as God designed.

When we purposefully allow ourselves to feel our feelings and surrender to the tears that may flow out, we experience a freeing and healing "release" that lessens our false perception that our feelings are too big and too scary.

By praying, we're inviting, welcoming, and receiving His healing as only He can heal, for He is at work in all things for our good.

Let's bring in the human experts:

> In addition to being self-soothing, shedding emotional tears releases oxytocin and endorphins.

> These chemicals make people feel good and may also ease both physical and emotional pain. In this way, crying can help reduce pain and promote a sense of well-being.[13]

The excerpt is from an article titled "Eight benefits of crying: Why it's good to shed a few tears." The biblical meaning of the number eight is known as *new beginnings*. Isn't that what we allow when we feel our feelings and let those flow out with a good cry? That's an interesting phrase, "a good cry." Have you ever cried so long and hard that the crying transformed into laughter? Crying is transformative.

One of the eight benefits in the article is "releases toxins and relieves stress. . . . [T]ears contain a number of stress hormones."[14] Isn't God's creation of our bodies stunningly miraculous?

Feeling our feelings is good; God created us to feel our emotions for many reasons, including our transformation.

If you're well-practiced in not feeling, you can renew your mind to intentionally practice feeling and expressing your feelings:

- First to God.
- Perhaps also to a trusted individual. Who is your human confidant? If you haven't yet sought out or found an individual whose lifestyle and mindset reflects Jesus, a good starting place is among your church family and those who are dedicated to a life unbinged, yoked with Christ.
- Write, write, write! The physical act of handwriting is also a form of emotional

release. Be honest in your writing. You can even direct your writing to God. *Dear Father, I feel . . .* If you're uncomfortable writing because someone might see and read your private thoughts, consider turning your written pages into an offering to God. Shred your handwritten pages and consider safely burning the strips, just as Christ "gave himself up for us as a fragrant offering and sacrifice" (Ephesians 5:2). Or plant the strips in your garden or pots as a symbol of your total surrender to Christ, fully enveloped in Him and growing in Him.

> *We can release all of our feelings at the feet of Jesus!*

"He heals the brokenhearted and binds up their wounds" (Psalm 147:3). Jesus is our great physician (Mark 2:17). But just as we must take action to visit our medical doctors, we must take action to go to the greatest physician, Jesus. No appointment needed; totally free and available 24/7!

Emotions Wheel

Another resource I love is the emotions wheel below. The wheel enables you to zero in on specific emotions rather than those that identify a broad category of emotions.

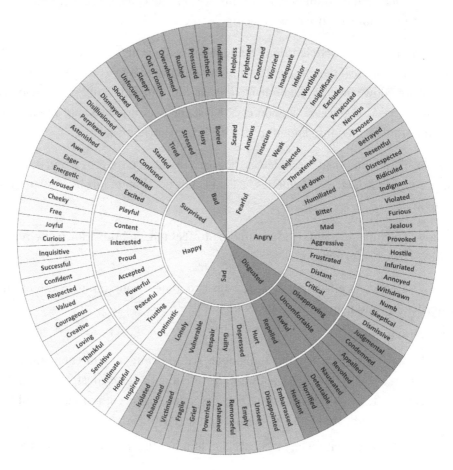

Let's begin at the center of the wheel: angry, disgusted, sad, happy, surprised, and bad. Let's say you're feeling sad, but you don't know why. On a piece of paper or in your journal, write:

> I feel sad.

Then dig deeper to uncover why you feel sad by looking at this next ring, the section beyond "Sad," and read each emotion: hurt, depressed, guilty, etc. Note from that section the emotion(s) that resonates with you. For example, let's say that *hurt* identifies or further explains your sadness. Write, "I feel hurt." Your writing will begin to form a visual shape:

> I feel sad.
>
> I feel hurt.

Who hurt me? Write their first name or their relationship to you.

> I feel sad.
>
> I feel hurt. —the committee vice president.

Move to the outer circle of the "Sad" section to identify your other feelings. Let's say you also feel embarrassed, disappointed, and victimized. Write those down.

> I feel sad.
>
> I feel hurt. —the committee vice president
>
> I feel embarrassed, disappointed, and victimized.

You feel really disappointed in the committee vice president you serve alongside. She made a poor choice against you. She got the facts mixed up and gossiped an untruth about you, making you feel victimized and embarrassed.

Next, study the entire wheel to discover other feelings you're experiencing. You realize you also feel betrayed, which you found in the wheel's zone beyond "Angry." You feel betrayed and angry by the circumstance, so write that down.

> I feel sad.
>
> I feel hurt. —the committee vice president
>
> I feel embarrassed, disappointed, and victimized.
>
> I feel betrayed and angry.

And so forth.

If you keep searching the wheel, you may eventually discover that this search has moved you into the "Surprised" zone. You may be amazed by all that you've uncovered. Plus, you may be in awe of God as the Potter who shaped you and equipped you to return to Him.

> I feel sad.
>> I feel hurt. —the committee vice president
>>> I feel embarrassed, disappointed, and victimized.
>>>> I feel betrayed and angry.
>>>> I feel amazed and awed by my discoveries.

Those feelings may land you in the "Happy" zone of the wheel, glad to have released all the yuckiness and now feeling peaceful. Perhaps you'll then feel accepting again that everyone is imperfect and will fail. You may then feel free and also thankful to God for the transformative discovery journey.

> I feel sad.
>> I feel hurt. —the committee vice president
>>> I feel embarrassed, disappointed, and victimized.
>>>> I feel betrayed and angry.
>>>> I feel surprised and amazed by my discoveries.
>>>>> I feel peaceful, accepting, free, and thankful.

As you see, the wheel helps to open the valve of your emotions to allow all the yucky feelings to stream out onto the paper and into God's ears—and even to free and renew you.

"Peace I Leave with You" (John 14:27)

When Jesus ascended into heaven, He gifted us with His divine peace and Holy Spirit. He knew we would need His ongoing presence; His supernatural comfort in times of disappointment, hurt, and grief; His calm in times of anxiety and fear; His guidance and direction in times of confusion and questions; His clarity and strength in times of temptation; His Word, which is God Himself; His assurance and faith that He loves us and will never leave us nor forsake us; and His grace and peace.

As you've seen here and experienced in your walk with Christ, knowing and trusting in all of who God is can't help but reveal His peace in us, regardless of the circumstance. His abiding Spirit provides everything we need to be our imperfect best for His glory.

Action Step: Mindset Matters

How we think (mindset) and what we choose to think about as we move through our various circumstances can bury God's gift of peace. His peace doesn't depart from us; we depart from His peace. Consider how these examples relate in you:

- You may be carrying miserable emotions from childhood, and living with those may be your uncomfortably comfortable state of resignation.

- Worries, anxieties, and fears from big events—even the happy ones like marriage and birthing babies—may have taken up residence in you like a handful of clouds that remain over you. Maybe you've grown so accustomed to sharing space with these emotions that you no longer see them for what they truly are: peace stealers.

- Those same emotions likely rise in you as you anticipate upcoming encounters like potlucks, birthday parties, and holiday dinners, and you allow those robbers to stay in you, perhaps out of habit.

1. Spend time uncovering all your worries, anxieties, and fears, and list those in the left-hand column.

Worries/Anxieties/Fears	Truth/Comfort

2. Now, in the right-hand column, write the promise from Jesus found in John 20:19: *Peace be with you.* On <u>each line</u> of your list, write those four powerful words of divine promise. In other words, no ditto marks! You're doing transformative work, renewing your mind. So carry that promise with you throughout your days.

I want you to know God's grace and peace throughout every day, in every circumstance. Keeping your heart and mind bathed in God's promises is an act of receiving His all.

Let's practice surrendering our all to Christ and receiving His all.

> "The Lord bless you
> and keep you;
> the Lord make his face shine on you
> and be gracious to you;
> the Lord turn his face toward you
> and give you peace."
>
> (Numbers 6:24–26)

CHAPTER 23

Grace upon Grace

OUR STRUGGLE IS WITH OUR COMMITMENT TO STAY ON PLAN IN DAILY LIFE AND DURING THE OCCASIONAL BIG EVENTS. Even when we're diligent to stay focused on eating compliantly and we're steadfast in watching out for the enemy and danger zones, life is hard, as Jesus said it would be (John 16:33). But in His great love and mercy, He gave us an amazing provision: grace.

Merriam-Webster nailed the definition of grace: "unmerited divine assistance given to humans for their regeneration or sanctification."[15] In other words, grace is God's *help* and *love* to humans that we don't deserve and cannot earn. God gives us grace to help us better ourselves and our lives.

The problem is that we don't typically *live in* grace upon grace, truly receiving it and applying it to ourselves and our circumstances.

Grace is even more elusive when we're addicted to a specific sin, like overeating. Although overeating seems harmless at first, it can quickly become a sin problem. Even at our best, we will fall into a mess of our own making because we're not perfect and never will be this side of heaven. God knew our sin nature before creating us, which is why—out of His great love, mercy, and grace for us—He planned to give His Son's life for our redemption. Jesus became the solid, immovable bridge of *grace* (favor) over our sin nature so we could go directly and boldly to our holy Father's throne, just as we are.

> From his fullness we have all received, grace upon grace already given. (John 1:16 ESV)

Does grace upon grace excuse us to continue in willful sin? No, for willfully sinning is not righteousness (right living). But just as we have God's forgiveness, we have the power of His grace to (1) accept ourselves as human, as He does, and not enter into self-sabotaging thoughts and (2) push forward through the tough times when our defenses are put to a greater test, such as during and after big events. We are to use the power of His grace to *overcome temptation* rather than to excuse willful sinning. As the apostle Paul taught new believers, he made these points:

> Shall we go on sinning so that grace may increase? By no means! We are those who have died to sin; how can we live in it any longer? . . . For sin shall no longer be your master, because you are not under the law, but under grace. (Romans 6:1–2, 14)

So here's the defining question regarding our overeating sin and all others:

> If the grace of Jesus Christ is "sufficient" (the solid rock bridge between us and God the Father), and grace is His nature extended to us in sufficiency, and if we are to be like Christ, then why would we not logically extend that same grace to ourselves across every aspect of our lives?

Sit with that truth.

God extends grace upon grace for all our needs and for every step and misstep. But it's up to each of us to choose and use His grace power toward ourselves, right living, and others.

Living Proactively vs. Reactively

Daily life and big events present temptations, like overeating and otherwise moving off the food plan: weddings, births, holiday gatherings, vacations. And on the other end of life's spectrum is loss. The loss of loved ones by way of death, broken relationships, divorce, a job that moves us away from loved ones, job losses, injuries, accidents, illnesses, and natural and economic hits and disasters all increase the addict's temptation to give in and give up. And in between the two extremes is our everyday life.

How do we best manage daily life and our readiness for big events and recovery? By proactively walking with Jesus and practicing grace toward ourselves. We must have a strategic plan, stay organized, and remain determined to follow through. Whatever we practice on a daily basis is what we will do during life's big events, affecting our recovery phase.

God, in His grace, gave us all the tools we need to *best* motor through daily life, big events, the expected and unexpected, and recovery. But are we choosing to remain filled with grace power as a daily practice to ensure successful motoring through and optimal recovery? In other words, are we living daily life proactively to ensure we remain grace-fueled, or are we living reactively to life's day-to-day and big events? If there is any uncertainty, spend time answering these questions:

1. Do I typically move through my days, big events, and recovery

   - proactively—staying filled with God's grace, applying that grace toward myself, even when I misstep (human nature), strategically planning, staying organized, and following through

     or

   - reactively—grabbing hold of the closest emotional ledge and hoping to hang on?

2. With those choices in mind, what degree of grace do I allow myself to move through daily life, big events, missteps, ditch dives, and recovery? 100 percent grace? 50 percent, 20 percent, or less?

3. On the grace scale—10 being grace upon grace and 1 being no grace—what level of grace do I grant myself in planning, organizing, and following through?

4. When I reach the other side of a normal day and a big event, do I typically

   - move into and through recovery in well-strengthened grace

     or

   - crash and burn in some way (mentally, physically, emotionally, spiritually), low on willpower to take the next right steps?

After a hard or exhilarating day or event, you've likely noticed a sense of letdown or a full-on crash and burn. Lack of energy to engage willpower is as normal as your vehicle running low (or empty) of fuel. So the point here is how well-prepared you are for recovery.

Grace Recovery and Zebras

Imagine a herd of graceful zebras running at top speed, fueled by adrenaline, through lion territory. What we know about zebras is that their journey through life is strikingly similar to ours.

- Zebras are constantly on the move through various environments. Like us, they are no strangers to parched, dry, and often unforgiving environments of constant threats. (Sound familiar?)
- Their exhilarating big events include rivers of fresh water (rare), lush fields of fresh grass (rare), and events like their babies' births. (All sound familiar?)
- Their terrifying big events include moving through lion territory, avoiding poachers, and staying safe through natural disasters. (Sound familiar?)

Here's where we tend to part ways from the zebras' lifestyle of grace for themselves and others:

- Zebras continually search for refueling (fresh grass and water). They know, value, and seek what's healthy—premium fuel—and avoid what's unhealthy.
- They're constantly on watch for enemies and hazards. Their eyes and ears are always alert. Even while resting, zebras extend the grace of watchfulness to themselves and their loved ones.
- Zebras strategize, plan, stay organized, and remain together in community support to optimize their well-being through their journeys and recoveries.
- They take intervals throughout the day, every day, to rest and refuel, resetting their ability to power through the next leg of the journey, whatever that will bring, the big events of joys and threats.

In contrast, we tend to find it difficult to move through and recover well (grace abounding) from a hard or exhilarating day and life's big events. Why? Because we don't consistently practice *daily grace habits*—a grace-upon-grace lifestyle. We lack grace for ourselves, which results in a collapse and a lack of grace toward others.

While we can plan for many events, life surprises us with unplanned happenings, primarily devastating. Our daily practices (habits) will set us up for either *reactive collapse* or *proactive recovery*.

Reactive living is to dismiss God's gifts of grace.

We can't help but live reactively when we have no specific meal plans in place, no recovery plan mapped out, and no daily intervals of *grace pauses* to rest and refuel our willpower with grace power. The results are (1) poor decisions, (2) falling into the enemy's traps, (3) relapsing into our addictions, (4) collapsing, and (5) lack of quality recovery.

Proactive living is to be yoked with Christ, continually refueled by God's grace.

Choosing to live proactively means staying engaged in strategic planning and organization, practicing daily intervals of *grace pauses* that sufficiently refuel us to take the next right steps through the remainder of the day. Proactive living prepares us for future big events, known and unknown, and thereby we recover well.

> **Refueled by His grace**, what were once deserts, "He makes me lie down in green pastures, he leads me beside still waters, he refreshes my soul" (Psalm 23:1–3).

> **Refueled by His grace**, what were once arduous mountains, "He guides me along the right paths [strategic and planned] for his name's sake" (Psalm 23:3, author addition).

> **Refueled by His grace**, "even though I walk through the darkest valley, I will fear no evil [food temptations and traps], for you are with me; your rod and your staff, they comfort me [His presence, grace, and protection]" (Psalm 23:4, author addition).

> **Refueled by His grace**, we can mentally, practically, and prayerfully anticipate and plan for recovery, knowing that recovery can be difficult.

But do we anticipate and plan for the enemy's enticements like this one?

> "Girl, look what you just made it through! Go ahead; you've earned that extra helping *and* a dessert—just this once. That's *real* grace for yourself!"

We fall into his trap of skewed thoughts and end up confusing *grace* with *entitlement*. Even when we've just taken the next right step, we can fall from grace (so to speak) with twisted self-talk:

> "Whoo-hoo, look what I just did! I made it through the day without moving off my food plan—*and* I got through everything gracefully. I deserve a reward—just this once."

Don't confuse grace with thinking you're *entitled* to a meal off-plan or a day off from clear-minded thinking through your food choices.

Never is it a good idea to take a meal or a day off from your food plan.

One willful decision outside of God's grace protection can be fatal to those of us who are dealing with addiction. One willful misstep doesn't simply weaken our defenses but slays our resolve to take the next right step. For most food addicts, one bite, one meal, or one day off the food plan plunges them into days of bingeing. It then takes tremendous effort, time, and energy (though depleted) to detox while also maneuvering through traps continually set by the roaring lion.

> **Refueled by His grace**, we can confidently say, "You prepare a table before me in the presence of my enemies [food of God's best when surrounded by unhealthy foods and temptation]. You anoint my head with oil [His blessings]; my cup overflows [peace, joy, contentment, . . .]" (Psalm 23:4–5, author addition).

Plan for recovery!

Strategies to Ensure You're Prepped and Ready for Grace-Filled Recovery

Think of all the planning that goes into a vacation: where you're going, what you'll eat, how much money you'll need to save toward vacation spending, where you'll stay, what you'll need to pack, etc.

Why do we maneuver attentively and strategically through all of these aspects? So we'll have the best vacation! Likewise, for the best recoveries and reentries, you must practice grace upon grace upon grace, day in and day out, and give as much planning to those as you give to planning your days and big events. Doing so will reserve your willpower to recover well from unexpected hard days and big events and to reenter the next leg of your journey strong.

Post-Trip Recovery Tips

- Plan your meals in advance for the day you'll arrive back home.
- Without planning, you're more likely to walk in the door and make regretful food choices, which will suddenly and surely steal the remnants of joy you carried home from your trip. Such a domino effect of loss will quickly move you from a letdown into a breakdown.
- The following grace strategy options may create for you a smoother transition back into normal life after vacation:

  Option 1: Plan to eat your first meal at a restaurant. Not Mexican, where chips and salsa automatically appear in front of you.

  Option 2: Get takeout from a restaurant you know has a compliant meal you can choose.

Option 3: Order from your local grocery store a compliant deli meal or compliant groceries for curbside pickup. That's my favorite plan, and a lifesaver for me. With curbside, I'm not in the enemy aisles with noncompliant foods staring at me. While guarded inside my vehicle, I can order produce, meats, and other compliant foods.

Maybe you're concerned about reentry costs, having just spent money on your vacation. Consider this: There's a substantially greater cost emotionally, mentally, and physically in eating off-plan than in a few extra dollars spent to safeguard staying on plan.

- Grace pace yourself back into day-to-day life.

You don't have to tackle all the reentry tasks in one day. Know this:

Small successes create significant successes.

You'll maximize a successful reentry if you limit your tasks to these three:
1. eating well
2. providing for your family
3. taking a nap or attending a pre-scheduled pampering appointment (manicure, pedicure, massage)

- Schedule ahead the grace time you need for self-care and easing into your normal routine. For example, don't make any appointments for the Monday after a big weekend or for the day after a big holiday or vacation. No appointment unless it's for grace pampering.

Grace does not carry guilt.

Unpacking your luggage and otherwise hitting the ground running can wait a few days. Before reentry, set your mind against allowing the enemy to steal your grace with the twisted idea that you have to do everything on the first day or even in the first week back home.

He'll say, "You have so much you need to get done that you better get started now!" His twisted thinking is an invitation to willfully or accidentally take a misstep instead of taking the next right steps.

Think of this "fall from grace" as falling down a staircase. You're standing on the top landing, "high" from your vacation (or another event), facing the entire staircase of steps back to normal life. Naturally, you can become overwhelmed and risk a misstep that will send you tumbling quickly, painfully, and dangerously to the bottom: bingeing.

It's perfectly okay to take some days to get back to your normal, healthy grace routine. Reentry isn't easy, so give yourself grace upon grace with wise, non-food rewards.

Grace Time to Rest and Reset

Typically, there are particular times of day when we struggle the most to stay true to a life unbinged. Most people say afternoon, around three or four o'clock, and again after dinner, around eight or nine. Those are my two most challenging times. Sometimes I'll go through a period of struggling every afternoon. Other times, food calls my name late in the evening and I'll struggle.

What about you? What times of day are hardest for you? As you consider that, think back to what you read about willpower, the Holy Spirit, and the importance of pausing to rest and reset.

**Struggles are more challenging when we allow the fuel
of willpower to run low or completely out.**

Would you continue to drive your vehicle with the gauge near or on empty? How much more important are your body, mind, emotions, and spirit?

Let's stay full by remaining connected to our premium fuel source, Jesus Christ. And when we make a misstep that can lead to bingeing, let's remember and take these essential next right steps:

- Turn to God—not in shame but in honesty.

- Identify the why. What were your first thought, first feeling, and first circumstance that led you to turn from God's best?

- Learn from the why. What safeguard will you put in place to avoid those "firsts"? Avoiding life isn't the answer; rather, it is how you navigate through various circumstances.

- Move forward with the knowledge and imagery that you are fully wrapped in His grace, thereby extending grace to yourself with a heart of true commitment to stay within the boundaries of God's best for you.

Give yourself grace upon grace upon grace.

Action Step: My Daily Rest and Reset Plan

Part of the grace-upon-grace lifestyle is taking a daily *rest and reset* time to refuel your willpower.

1. Choose a reset time.

    Mine is three o'clock in the afternoon. My phone alarm is set to remind me to pause, rest, and reset. I encourage you to set a reminder that's most effective in getting your attention. You may need to change the means occasionally because we grow so accustomed to repetition that we no longer hear it, see it, or feel it.

2. Decide how much reset time you need for each interval.

    I need approximately five to ten minutes. We're each different. Maybe you need ten or twenty minutes.

3. Create and commit to your daily rest and reset plan—the when, where, and what.

    Let's say your struggle begins at about 3:00 p.m. each day, and you need ten minutes to pause, rest, and reset. Where do you plan to go, and what do you plan to do?

    Examples:

    Where

    -   Go outside to a peaceful area.
    -   At home, you may prefer your prayer closet or favorite quiet room. (The bathroom counts!)
    -   At work and church, you may want to go into the supply closet, an empty office, or an unused conference room.
    -   At a big event, walk until you find a place of quiet and solitude.

    What

    -   Pray.
    -   Recite the Scripture verses you've memorized.
    -   Pick up where you left off in reading your Bible. (For away times, there are purse-size Bibles and Bible apps for your phone.)
    -   Sing or listen to praise and worship songs, or perhaps you're a musician and will want to strum your guitar or play the piano.
    -   Dance.
    -   Lie on the floor, looking toward the heavens, imagining yourself resting in the arms of God.

When I hear my reminder at three o'clock, I take a few minutes to finish what I'm doing, and then I typically grab sparkling water or a cup of coffee or tea and go outside. I pray, "Lord, I just need to take this time with You." I read a bit of Scripture and sometimes listen to a worship song.

Whatever you need to do to practice the daily grace of resting, resetting, and refueling your willpower, plan it and do it. Make your grace time a priority and keep it fresh by changing the plan as needed.

4. Below, set your daily pause time(s). You may need two occasionally or each day.

Pause Time: _____ Pause Time: _____

Pause Length: _____ mins.

5. Set a reminder(s) on your phone or whatever device will alert you to pause.

6. Set your pause locations below. Include more than one to allow for variable circumstances (like weather, if you like to be outdoors) and for mixing things up.

_____   _____

_____   _____

7. Set your pause time activities.

_____   _____

_____   _____

8. If you love music, prepare your playlist now.

CHAPTER 24

Raising Kids in a Sugar-Obsessed World

SUGAR IS IN EVERYTHING, AND SUGARY FOODS ARE EVERYWHERE! Growing up, I knew I had a problem with sugar and flour, eating bagged and packaged processed foods. But when I became a mom, the sugar popularity really got my attention.

I remember running errands with my toddler in tow, and almost everywhere we stopped, an employee gave my daughter a cookie, a mint, or a lollipop. She wasn't even two yet! I was so upset. *How am I going to raise my children differently than I was raised so they won't have a sugar and flour obsession?*

I did not want my kids to endure long-term suffering as I had. But I didn't have a solution at that time. I simply did everything possible to avoid exposing them to unhealthy foods and eating patterns. Food as rewards, bribes, or soothing was not in the picture. I was determined to raise my children very differently than I'd been raised regarding food. Still, I didn't have the exact answer on how to pull that off since I was in the throes of food addiction. I only knew I had to protect my children and that *something* had to change.

My favorite Scriptures that speak to generational change are in 1 Kings and 2 Kings:

> Elijah went before the people and said, "How long will you waver between two opinions? If the Lord is God, follow him; but if Baal is God, follow him." But the people said nothing. (1 Kings 18:21)

Do we serve God or Baal? What are we going to do? They wavered, not wanting to decide.

Fast forward to 2 Kings 17:41.

> Even while these people were worshiping the Lord, they were serving their idols. To this day their children and grandchildren continue to do as their ancestors did.

Their parents hadn't created a new path for them.

Today and every day after, you and I get to choose who we will serve: ourselves or God, our idols or God, traditions or God—whether we're wrestling food issues, other idols, or generational chains. The thought that we can change the course for future generations is powerful. Sit with that truth. No matter our present stage or age, who and what we commit to and stick to will influence the younger generation and those to come.

Feeding Tips

No matter what children you influence (your own or others), the following feeding tips are for you. By following these Stop, Set, Stick-To, and Stay tips, you're showing favor (grace) and love to everyone under your care, observing you, and to yourself.

- Stop using food as a reward, bribe, or soother.
- Set an eating schedule for your family and yourself.
- Stick to your mission of doing the next right thing.
- Stay within the boundaries.

Before I changed my food lifestyle, I made double batches of my favorite dessert and hid a batch just for me that my family didn't know about. I'd be in and out of the freezer, grabbing the extras whenever I wanted a hand-to-mouth comfort fix.

Destructive.

I no longer make double batches, which was a double foothold, one for Satan against me and one for me against myself. My plan now includes the many sugar-free and flour-free recipes I've gathered and created.

For special occasions and traditions, I still bake cookies with my kids and even bake their birthday cakes, but now I stick to my mission and stay within my food boundaries.

I did a little experiment with my kids that demonstrated a powerful lesson about temptation. I set out a jar of cookies, and sure enough, what happened when they saw the cookies? They wanted a cookie. After a time, I put the cookies out of sight in a pantry drawer. Guess what? Nobody thought about cookies. Out of sight, out of mind. When we see something that tempts us, we're more inclined to want that item, just like looking at a toy catalog. Oh my goodness! They "need" a lot of stuff after looking at a toy catalog, brightly displayed toys they hadn't known existed.

Out of sight, out of temptation.

Stock Food Carefully

The same experiment outcome applies to stocking up on food. People stock up for different reasons. We saw this when the pandemic hit, as we do when a winter storm is forecasted. Some people stay stocked up "just in case" something might happen, and others stock up because they don't like shopping. Whatever the case, we food addicts need to be very cautious about *what* we stock up on because we don't want to put ourselves in a position that invites a binge.

I generally keep very little processed food in our house. I have Costco-size boxes of healthy granola bars for my family, but I must be very cautious because a granola bar is one of my "gateway" foods—a binge waiting to happen. Even though the item is healthy by serving size, the sweet hint in a granola bar draws me into eating for pleasure and wanting more.

I make sure my family knows that the granola bars are there, and I say, "Those are not for me; they're for you, and this is how much is there." The verbalized statement is a good safety net for me because I'm the one who's tempted to binge.

- The verbalization says this to my brain: *Those items are not yours!*
- The verbalization establishes accountability for me, so I'm less likely to dip in and eat.

Set a Food Routine

Setting a meal routine for our families is one of the greatest gifts we can give our children and ourselves. Creating *set* mealtimes gives children security around food, establishes healthy boundaries, and cultivates the grace of occasionally feeling hungry between meals. Plus, feeding kids all day is exhausting, and when snacks are served at all times, temptations abound for us to eat off-plan and for them to eat more than they need.

The specifics of your children's daily meal routine will be unique to your family. Some will do fine with three meals and one snack. Others may need three meals and three snacks. The number of eating times isn't as important as the fact that these are *structured times* for your child to have access to delicious, healthy food.

As an example, here's a meal routine our family has followed:

> 8:00 a.m. – breakfast
> 11:30 a.m. – lunch instead of a mid-morning snack
> 3:00 p.m. – snack for my children (the one and only snack)
> 6:00 p.m. – family dinner

Regarding my children's afternoon snack (if they're hungry), they get to choose a fruit or vegetable and a protein. Healthy snacks! Examples: apple and peanut butter or string cheese and carrots.

Here's the hunger test: If they're truly hungry, they'll enjoy those foods. If they want to eat for the sake of eating rather than actual hunger, they'll want a bag of chips, for example.

For dinner, we enjoy a nice, big, healthy meal, and the children decide when they're finished eating. They know that our kitchen is closed after dinner and that breakfast is coming. So even if someone is hungry before bedtime, they know that's okay because breakfast will come. Also, our family doesn't eat dessert most nights. When we do, it's pre-scheduled into the meal plan.

Our rule: No getting into our fridge or pantry after dinner. Why? People get into the most eating trouble after dinner. Think about your evenings. Maybe the kids are in bed, the work is done, nobody's around to see your activities or see you as their example, and food calls out to you.

We've become a hand-to-mouth comfort culture. Fast food delivery is at an all-time high, and food is readily available a few feet from the recliner and big-screen TV. Our homes morph into movie theaters that tell us the experience will be better if we're also entertained by food.

Destructive.

Perhaps your evening scenes are not so cozy because you're battling past or present turbulent circumstances that eat away at your mind and heart. In munching, you find emotional comfort and distraction, a means to stuff those thoughts and feelings deeper.

Destructive.

Close the kitchen after dinner. Exceptions:

- **If you have a baby**, obviously they need to nurse or bottle-feed on their schedule, which gradually changes as they move through the various growth stages.

- **If you have a toddler**, they will need to eat more often because they have tiny tummies and their bodies are in full-force growth mode—a natural process that you and I have long surpassed, yet we continue to yield to. As children move into self-feeding, you're setting the stage for their future eating patterns. So taking the next right step is not exclusive to you; it includes feeding your family nutritiously, at healthy intervals, while teaching them about food health and moderation. We can talk to our children continuously about health, but like a megaphone, our actions speak louder than our words.

- **If you have a child with special needs, ADHD, or past trauma**, they may need a different meal structure or more support around mealtimes. I encourage you to talk to your doctor or therapist about the best feeding practices for your particular child's needs. It's possible to accommodate all kinds of circumstances while being intentional about how your children are fed.

- **If you have older children or teenagers**, set a family meal structure that works for everyone. Enlist their help in the kitchen preparing healthy snacks and meals for the family. Focus on progress over perfection and ease their way into healthier eating habits.

Grace doesn't mean getting everything we want when we want it.

Grace means favoring our families and ourselves so much (as God favors us) that we want only His best: health, patience, gratitude, and enjoyment of His gifts from the earth at the proper time and in moderation.

By allowing our children to eat and snack all day and evening (even healthy foods), we're not giving their bodies favorable (grace) opportunities to feel the *gifts* of hunger and anticipation of God's gracious food provision.

Yes, hunger and anticipation are grace gifts from God. Most of us in the US do not even darken the door of true hunger. Our kids should know a measure of hunger and the practice of patience while waiting for the next meal. Sometimes, my son would come home from school close to dinnertime and want to reach for a snack and I'd say cheerfully, "Dinner is coming soon!" The extra benefit of children experiencing growling tummies and meal anticipation is the likelihood that they'll eat the healthy foods on their plates and feel appreciative because they're more than ready for the meal. Triple win!

*There's nothing wrong with feeling hunger
and practicing patience.*

Part of being transformed by renewing our minds is letting go of lies like "I'm depriving my child" and feeling guilty. Think of it this way: When we allow our kids and ourselves to eat, eat, eat all day, even healthy foods, we're depriving them and ourselves of the grace gifts of food anticipation and appreciation.

Back to those occasional family desserts. . . . We have a special Sunday night dessert. My family doesn't miss dessert during the week because they're not accustomed to having it, except on Sunday evenings. The extra fun part is that my kids take turns making the Sunday dessert, presenting it to the family, and enjoying that time together. Sunday evening dessert is also a time for my kids to learn the ins and outs of the kitchen, venturing out of their comfort zones, learning about food preparation, cooking, and serving. The activity brings us all together for a fun tradition in moderation—only once a week. Even though it's only once a week, I choose to abstain from eating the dessert because it only makes me want more; and rather than being focused on the sweets, I want to be present with my family.

The Greatest Tip

I view the following tip as the greatest because I feel that the Lord allowed a light to shine on this one for me. I have one son and four daughters. My son played football, and we had a great time watching him. We were enjoying a game when one of the girls asked, "Can we go get a treat?"

I responded favorably, "We'll get a treat at halftime." In that moment, I had what felt like an epiphany. I said, "You know what, we're not going to get a 'treat' at halftime; we're going to get candy!" Oh, their faces! "You can have candy, but the 'treat' we're getting is sitting here together, having fun as a family, cuddled up, watching your brother play football, and laughing together. This is our treat."

I'd had this realization:

*A true treat is something we can hold onto
for the rest of our lives.*

I told the girls, "We're not going to call candy and other sweets a treat anymore because sweets are simply sugar. The real treat is the special time we spend together, creating lasting memories."

I encourage you to switch the food term "treat" to "sweet" and save "treat" for what it is: all the special times with those you love.

Final Tip: Sugar Points

Occasionally, our family has a fun competition we call sugar points. My friend Amy shared this with me and we love it. We'll pick a month, say February, and the kids agree on the number of sugar points they'll each have for that month. Let's say the agreed-upon number is ten, which means each kid can have a sugary food, if they want, up to ten times in February. Each time a kid has a sweet food, they note it on their chart as having used one sugar point. At the end of the month, the kid with the most remaining sugar points gets a non-food reward. (Our Sunday evening family desserts were freebies.)

Most importantly, this occasion helps them learn, understand, and practice budgeting, planning, and strategizing. They also see the benefit of saving—important knowledge they'll need to use when they're grown. If a kid chooses to eat their ten sweets in one week, fine. But then they're out of points for the rest of the month (and out of the running for the reward). So, for example, if there's a birthday party coming up in the chosen month, they'll want to make sure they have points to spend on the birthday cake and any candies in the typical take-home bag.

We all know that budgeting, planning, strategizing, and balancing between fun and responsibilities come into play in every aspect of our lives. Examples are time, energy, and money. The same principle applies to our essential need to plan and budget our food choices and portions and strategize for big events.

Excess adversely affects our mental, emotional, physical, and spiritual health. These four components are so tightly interconnected that when our body, for example, is unhealthy, our mental, emotional, and spiritual well-being is also harmed or, at least, threatened, depending on the degree of excess. Likewise, feeding our minds unhealthy material threatens our mental well-being, which affects our emotions, spirits, and even our bodies because emotions play an enormous role in how we physically feel. Add to that our propensity for emotional eating.

Our children and grandchildren need to see and learn from early in life how much and what foods they're consuming, just like monitoring what their mind is feeding on and the interconnected natural consequences. As for food, they need to understand why sugar, flour, and other processed-food limits are essential: because those choices can and do negatively affect their body and, in turn, their mind, emotions, and spirit.

We aren't just talking heads demanding, "Do as I say." We're behavioral examples.

Consider sugar points as a fun tool for your children or grandchildren. A lot of grandparents have a cookie jar, and some have sodas in the fridge. My parents and in-laws really enjoy "sweeting" their grandchildren—a fun part of grandparenting for many. Still, we can set boundaries. My kids know they can have two sweets at their grandparents' house. They don't get free rein of the cookie jar, refrigerator, or pantry. There's just no need for that.

In our world of excessive flour, sugar, other processed foods, and fast foods, it's hard to raise healthy kids. But teaching them about these hazards and the healthy alternatives can be done in fun ways as you move through life together, talking with them and being the example.

Maybe our kids and grandkids won't have food issues as adults. Or maybe they will. But they'll have seen how we broke our food bondage chains. In the process, we're also teaching them about grace—favoring their God-created body, mind, emotions, and spirit, their responsibility to take good care of the "temple" God entrusted to them, and how to fully surrender to Him in every area of life. As we talk with them and show them by example in the course of day-to-day living, our children and grandchildren learn how to view God and revere Him as the highest and greatest and how to keep everything else where it needs to be, at His feet.

Action Step: My Relationship with Food

Write a letter to God regarding your relationship with food. Put everything at His feet in detail. Ask forgiveness for your willful stumbling, thank Him for His grace and love, share with Him your struggles and commitment, . . . Your Father cares about every detail of your life.

The physical act of handwriting the letter will impress more deeply on your heart and mind

- a posture of humility and reverence at your Father's feet,
- full surrender to Him, reliance on Him, and trust in Him,
- your need for His help, forgiveness, love, and grace, and
- that His grace is the favor you must also extend to yourself.

Open your letter with the name you call God. Examples: Father, Abba, Daddy, God, King, . . .

_____

_____

_____

_____

_____

_____

_____

_____

CHAPTER 25

Jesus Wants to Eat With You

Did you know that Jesus wants to eat with you, sit across the table from you, be beside you at every meal? He said to us, "Behold, I stand at the door and knock. If anyone hears my voice and opens the door, I will come in to him and eat with him, and he with me" (Revelation 3:20 ESV). What an invitation! Jesus wants to eat with you!

If I had formerly accepted His invitation, realizing He was always sitting with me in love and faithfulness, I would have felt ashamed of my eating habits at some meals. He's always with us, but since we don't physically see Him as the apostles and others did, we're sometimes so wrapped up in our desires that we forget He's present, loves us, and is full of grace toward us.

In my head at that time, I felt like I was alone and secretly eating, which was no secret to Jesus. Still, He loved me through those long, dark years of my addiction. Even after everything He's seen of me, He still wants to eat with me. How grateful I am to be one of God's daughters, an heir with Jesus! Isn't it mind-blowing to consider that the Creator of the heavens and earth—everything that was made—wants to eat with us? Every day. Every meal. Shouldn't we then want to eat meals that glorify Him at a table fit for the King and His children?

God has exemplary taste not only in the foods He created but also in finery. Just read the account of God's very specific instructions to Moses and the Israelites for building, fashioning, and designing the temple. The passage is utterly amazing. Here are a couple of sample scenes where God is speaking to Moses, whom He's wrapped in a cloud of His great glory:

> You are to receive the offering for me from everyone whose heart prompts them to give. These are the offerings you are to receive from them: gold, silver and bronze; blue, purple and scarlet yarn and fine linen; goat hair; ram skins dyed red and another type of durable leather; acacia wood; olive oil for the light; spices for the anointing oil and for the fragrant incense; and onyx stones and other gems to be mounted on the ephod and breastpiece. (Exodus 25:1–7)

Further along in the chapter, He dedicates an entire section to the table specifics. Here's a taste:

> Overlay it with pure gold and make a gold molding around it. Also make around it a rim a handbreadth wide and put a gold molding on the rim. Make four gold rings for the table and fasten them to the four corners, where the four legs are. . . . And make its plates and dishes of pure gold, as well as its pitchers and bowls for the pouring out of offerings. Put the bread of the Presence on this table to be before me at all times. (Exodus 25:22–26, 29–30)

Now, consider the esthetic and ambiance differences between these two scenarios:

- a drive-through meal, eating in the car, or bingeing on it at home from the paper bag

or

- sitting at a dressed table, set with a beautifully planned and prepared meal in all the glorious colors of God's design

Don't miss the point. Jesus ate with people in whatever their conditions and surroundings, and He loved each person, destitute or wealthy. Likewise, He graciously sits with us and loves us, whether we're bingeing from drive-through bags or dining from a well-dressed table of the freshest, healthiest foods. His *desire* for us is that every meal be His *finest*, the foods He created and was the first to plant for us. Imagine God's great love for us through His bountiful and breathtaking work of creation.

Wherever you are and in whatever condition, Your Father is with you and has already provided His finest foods. The next time you're at the grocery store, take a good, long look through the fresh produce and see—really see—each vibrant color and masterful shape. Then say to yourself, or aloud to your family member:

> *God made these beautiful foods for me because He loves me so much. Thank You, Lord! Thank You.*

Food and eating are beautiful gifts designed by God for our health and pleasure. But unfortunately, our world (each of us) has made quite the mess of meals: the vast range and supply *chains* (don't miss that pun) of addictive foods. The enemy cannot create or even begin to imitate God's finest, so he whispers in our ears about all sorts of special sauces and decorated desserts and pastries made from processed sugar and flour.

Our mistake is eating it. Our inner brokenness created a cavernous emotional need for comfort that we try to fill with processed foods, overeating, eating in excess, and bingeing.

Perhaps your brokenness is the result of traumatic situations. We each have different stories that led us to the same false answer: Food is emotional comfort and support. And Satan aways shows up to "help." He's the big bad wolf with all types of appealing disguises. Here are just a few examples:

- the grandma (Mrs. Smith, Mrs. Fields, Marie Callendar, . . .)
- the grandpa (Colonel Sanders, Papa John, . . .)
- the professional (Chef Boyardee, Oscar Mayer, Duncan Hines, . . .)
- the fun friend (Little Debbie, Ben & Jerry, Wendy, Jack, Arby, Ronald McDonald, . . .)
- the royalty (Burger King, Smoothie King, Dairy Queen, . . .)

He reels us in with one look into his picnic basket, one smell, one invitation, one bite— "just one."

But—praise God—"the one who is in you is greater than the one who is in the world" (1 John 4:4). We can pause before pulling anything from Satan's basket and ditching our food plans. We can turn around and turn to Christ, ask for His help, and ask ourselves these essential questions:

- Is this food healthy or overly processed?
- Is this food on my plan for today?
- Why do I want to eat it? Am I genuinely hungry? Am I bored or anxious?

The big question: Will each of my answers and actions glorify God?

He loves us so much that He wants us to eat His finest and in fellowship with Him.

Emergency Food Kit

When following a specific food plan, having an emergency food kit (EFK) available is very helpful. An EFK is a great backup plan, like having a first aid kit and extra diapers. An EFK is a nice food support for unexpected circumstances that intersect with your planned mealtime or planned foods. Examples:

- You're at an event, and there's nothing compliant for you to eat. You can still enjoy eating with others (from your EFK).

- You've made an unexpected trip to the hospital with a loved one or friend. The time frame intersects with a planned mealtime, and cafeteria food and snack machine foods are noncompliant.

- Your doctor's appointment lasts far longer than anticipated, preventing you from enjoying your planned mealtime.

- You have a flat tire and must pull to the side of the road, and your wait time rolls into and past your planned mealtime.

Choose healthy items for your EFK—nonperishable foods that can stay in your car, in your purse, and at the office. Be intentional about preparing fresh foods for when you'll be out and about. Your measurements might be a bit off, but when you're in a food emergency, you do what you need to for timely and healthy nourishment, which means planning ahead to have healthy and compliant foods on hand.

**Food is fuel and is needed at planned times to keep
your body and mind energized and clear.**

As an example, below is my list of emergency items.

Tip: pop-top cans omit the need for a can opener.

Proteins
- 2 oz. of nuts
- 2 oz. packet of peanut butter
- single-serving tuna pouch

Vegetables
- pop-top can of corn, easy to drain and eat
- pop-top can of green beans
- pop-top can of lentil vegetable soup—a protein and vegetables

Fruits
- pop-top can of pineapple tidbits or mandarin oranges in light juice (no added sugar), easy to drain and eat

Grains
- 1 oz. of oats
- 1 oz. rice cakes

Fats
- 0.5 oz. of nuts

Beverages
- water
- a favorite tea bag to give you a little burst of flavored energy
- lemon juice packets for your tea or water
  For times when you just don't want water, a teabag and lemon juice packet are refreshing blessings.

Other Items
- salad dressing packet for events that may not have compliant dressings
  Tip: a little water, lemon juice, or salsa added to your dressing makes it go further.
- plastic forks and napkins
- willpower, which honors God and commitment to the plan

These foods may not be among your favorites, and eating out of a can is not ideal, but you know it tastes better than nothing and certainly better than going off-plan. Plus, the items are nutritious, energizing, and compliant—having no sugar or flour.

**Remember, this kit is for emergencies and enables
you to stay within your boundaries.**

The Right Choice Is Always the Best Choice

Right choices don't always *feel* like the best choices in the moment. Sometimes, a quick hit of a particular food *feels* like it will make things better, which is why we tend to lean toward quick hits. We must put off temptations by turning from them to face Jesus. He is always there, offering His strength and a way of escape.

Turn from the temptations of quick hits. They are not God-honoring and offer no inherent reward. In fact, quick hits in the aftermath can be very painful physically, emotionally, mentally, and spiritually.

Rewards come from right choices, both in the moment and later.

I love how Galatians 6:9 reads so perfectly in the New King James Version: "Let us not grow weary while doing good, for in due season we shall reap if we do not lose heart." Isn't it easy to lose heart? It's also easy to think it's too hard to stand firm against quick hits and otherwise eating off-plan. We wonder why we make certain choices in one area but not others. I came across a beautifully written article emphasizing why we shouldn't take quick hits but rather make right choices. Here's an excerpt:

All temptation would be harmless . . . if sin promised no pleasure. . . . So the devil takes what fleeting pleasures there are in sin and makes them feel . . . sweeter than the pleasures at God's right hand. Our God-given desire for pleasure, forceful as the Niagara, cannot be dammed through mere self-denial. The river must run somewhere—and if not to sin, then to something better. [16]

The writer described a desperately thirsty hiker who denied himself a drink from a saltwater puddle because he knew there was a crystal stream just two miles farther on. The writer shared that we can "deny ourselves the easy and immediate for the difficult and delayed" in the same way the hiker did because we have knowledge that "God has supplied water far sweeter" if we "only keep walking with 'the assurance of things hoped for' (Hebrews 11:1)."[17]

When you desire food, wanting that immediate pleasure, think of that hiker and the saltwater. We want to pass that by for what's far sweeter and greater.

Action Step: Build Your Emergency Kit

1. Create your grocery list of emergency items.

2. You can make your kit even more fun by choosing a pretty insulated bag for your items.

_____

_____

_____

_____

_____

_____

_____

_____

_____

CHAPTER 26

Reaching and Maintaining Your Goal Body Range

Choosing Your Goal Body Range

OFTEN WE HAVE A SPECIFIC GOAL WEIGHT IN MIND, BUT LET'S CHANGE THAT TO "GOAL BODY" RANGE. Why? Although you may have a certain weight in mind, consider that as we age and change, that number may need to be adjusted. As you lose weight, you'll reach your goal body *range* that's indicated by these factors:

- My body feels good.
- My clothes fit well.
- I like what I see in the mirror.
- I feel comfortable with my size.

Surrender that range to God and ask Him for guidance. Choose your range based on those four factors and with the knowledge that you'll have weight ebbs and flows. Choosing your feel-good and look-good range allows for those fluctuations.

Commit to maintain your beautifully designed body by God, which He created specifically with you in mind for your joy and His glory.

The Maintenance Food Plan

As you near your goal body range, you'll move into determining how to maintain your goal. To ensure you'll remain successful in maintenance, slowly add compliant food. Knowing your body will change as you grow older, continue to be attentive to your body's unique needs; your body is the best communicator. Using the four bulleted indicators above, rather than just the scale, adjust your maintenance plan accordingly.

When to Add Additional Food

One of people's biggest fears when approaching maintenance is adding food. They feel great while on the weight loss plan, and they think that if they start adding food, they may start gaining weight again. I understand this fear. When you've worked so hard to lose weight, the LAST thing you want to do is gain it all back.

That possibility is why you must be proactive when transitioning to maintenance. As you get closer to your goal body, usually within 5–10 pounds, you may feel strong hunger and some mental food chatter leading up to mealtimes. That's a good sign that it's time to start adding food to your plan.

It might be tempting to wait until you get all the way down to your goal body weight to start adding food, but being proactive to add food sooner allows you to gently and slowly ease into your goal body. Making your first food addition doesn't mean you have to stop losing weight. It just means you're looking ahead and planning for maintenance. Imagine pulling your car off the highway into a parking lot. You don't keep going 55 mph until you find a parking spot. You slow down to pull in, and move carefully until you find the perfect place for you.

You can trust God with your maintenance food plan. If you make changes intentionally and prayerfully, He will guide you with all wisdom into the right amount of food to maintain your goal body.

What Servings to Add

As you move *gently* into maintenance, add the following foods in the order listed.

> **Very Important:** Add only *one* item and maintain that for *at least* one week before adding the next food. This gradual process (1) gives your body time to adjust and (2) allows you to see what your weight and body do before making the next addition.
>
> 1. Lunch—add 1 serving of grain
> 2. Breakfast—increase protein to 2 servings
> 3. Dinner—add 1 serving of grain

4. Lunch—increase protein to 2 servings
5. Dinner—add 1 serving of fruit

These food additions are typical for women. While most settle into their full maintenance by making 1–5 additions per day, the decision is based on what your unique body truly *needs* (not *desires*) to maintain your goal body. You may honestly need only one addition, or you may need three, for example.

Remember this: Additions are not about "I want to eat more" and fluctuating as you see fit. The boundary for additions is honesty in answering this question: "What does my body *need* to maintain my goal body?"

If you continue to lose weight after making the above additions, add food in the order listed below—one item and one week at a time.

1. Dinner—increase protein to 2 servings
2. Breakfast—increase grain to 2 servings
3. Lunch—increase fat to 2 servings
4. Dinner—increase fat to 2 servings
5. Lunch—increase grain to 2 servings

Surrendering Loose Skin

Once you've lost the excess weight, you'll likely have loose skin. This is an area of surrender that's so much easier than the food and weight-loss struggle that plagued you for so long.

Excess skin removal is a personal decision. There is no right or wrong. As always, ask God for His guidance.

Often skin tightens slightly as the weight is kept off for a period of time. So wait until after at least one year of food maintenance before deciding whether to have excess skin removed. You'll then have a clearer picture of what your body is going to look and feel like and you'll be in a better position to make that decision.

Surrendering the Number on the Scale

Most of us have a scale number we desire, whether as a goal or because that number will make us feel good. Maybe we'll get there; maybe not. Or perhaps we'll settle below the number.

Surrendering to God requires letting go of certain mindsets—that specific number on the scale being one of them.

In 2021, I was happily living in plan maintenance and at the goal weight I had set for myself. Everything was going well, and I was very pleased with the scale number. I watched that number remain steady for almost three years, never guessing it would change as long as I stayed within my food boundaries.

After a long battle with COVID, I ended up needing several infusions, as well as multiple chest x-rays. The results revealed a pneumomediastinum (in simple terms, an air pocket between my lungs) that required several rounds of heavy steroids. The drug caused an immediate weight gain. In addition, I wasn't able to taste or smell food. When those senses returned, my brain started demanding extremely salty foods. Let's just say I moved out of the maintenance goal I'd set for myself.

I have yet to return to that scale number, though I've maintained the 100-pound loss. I'm very pleased—except the scale number is higher than I'd hoped, even though I follow the food boundaries.

I try to focus on the factors that maintain my goal *body range* (explained at the beginning of this chapter) rather than solely on the scale number. Letting go of the number was another level of surrender, trust, and obedience that required me to "renew my mind." My focus is to continue eating within food boundaries; the weight will settle whenever it settles.

The Big Picture

There will be times when you'll want to go back to your old way of eating. Your brain may say, "Let's just stop weighing our food," or "We can eat whenever we want," or "Let's try moderation again." Giving in to such thoughts will easily get you off track and back into your old habits and patterns.

Remember the reasons the plan works:

- You're committed to this new path forward, leaving the old behind.
- You're surrendered to God and His best—no processed sugar, no flour.
- You're weighing and measuring food.
- You're maintaining success.

I love the phrase my good friend Noreen Savage says:

If you go back to your old WAYS,
you'll go back to your old WEIGHS.

You've come so far! An amazing, great distance. You've done the tough work, at times against great temptation and other struggles. **Celebrate! Give thanks!**

This forward journey is ongoing and will, like everything in life, have its physical, mental, and emotional challenges and spiritual warfare. Stay alert; the enemy doesn't want you to gain any more victories. But you've proven to him (and yourself) that you are more than a conqueror. You are an overcomer! So view this journey as a reminder that you *can* indeed do *all* things through Christ, who gives you strength!

Enjoy your healthy body, mind, and spirit to the fullest, maintaining this fresh and fit Christ-centered lifestyle, and view the remainder of your life's journey through His eyes and His distinctive purpose for you.

> You make known to me the path of life; you will fill me with joy in your presence, with eternal pleasures at your right hand. (Psalm 16:11)

We did it, and we can continue to live life unbinged. Together! Stay committed, connected, and refreshed alongside your life unbinged sisters.

Commit to living the rest of your days yoked with Christ, living fully and freely within the boundaries of God's best—the vast, flourishing, generous, vibrant garden of choices He lovingly, perfectly prepared *for you*!

Action Step: Enveloped in the Folds of God's Love

In the Psalm 23 paraphrase below, place your name within the folds of God's love as you read aloud, slowly and thoughtfully. Imagine yourself in your heavenly Father's arms, fully immersed in His love as it truly is: the most luxurious, refreshing, satisfying, peace-filled banquet and bath, attended by the Servant of all servants, your Savior, Jesus:

> The Lord is _____'s shepherd; she lacks nothing.
>
> He urges _____ to rest peacefully in His luxurious green pastures.
>
> He leads _____ beside tranquil waters and fully refreshes her soul.
>
> He guides _____ along the right paths for her greatest good, bringing glory to His name. . . .
>
> He prepares a luxurious and bountiful table for _____ in the presence of her enemies.
>
> He anoints _____'s head with oil, blessing her and setting her apart as His daughter; her cup overflows with everything she needs and more.
>
> Most certainly, the Lord's goodness and love will follow _____ all the days of her life, and she will dwell in complete love, peace, and joy in her Lord's house forever.

Now, read the passage again, believing with firm and full conviction that you *are* the daughter of the King of kings. Believe your Father's written thoughts to you. Allow the passage to fill the deepest recesses of your soul and overflow through all your days.

> The Lord *is* my shepherd; I lack *nothing.*
>> He urges me to *rest* peacefully in His luxurious green pastures.
>> He leads me beside tranquil waters and fully *refreshes* my soul.
>> He guides me along the *right* paths for my greatest good, bringing *glory to His name.* . . .
>> He prepares a luxurious and bountiful table for me in the presence of my enemies.
>> He anoints my head with healing oil, blessing me and setting me apart as His daughter; my cup *overflows* with *everything I need* and more.
>> Most certainly, the Lord's goodness and love *will* follow me *all the days of my life,* and I *will* dwell in complete love, peace, and joy in my Lord's house *forever.*

Bonus Online Content

Print a free Psalm 23 worksheet for yourself and to share with your daughters, granddaughters, sisters, mothers, and friends.

CONCLUSION

Accountability Group

WHEN I STARTED THE JOURNEY TO UNBINGE MY LIFE, I WAS
AWARE THAT MANY PEOPLE PARTICIPATE IN VARIOUS GROUPS FOR
ACCOUNTABILITY, SUPPORT, AND MASTERMINDING. I had a friend who
also wanted to live a life free of sugar and flour, and we really enjoyed talking about
our new lifestyle. We supported each other and even shared food plans, which was
super helpful. She was my accountability buddy.

Another friend suggested that I put together a mastermind accountability group. I
wasn't interested, primarily because I didn't want to be accountable to anyone. But
the seed she planted began to take root, and my thinking changed. Although I had a
buddy to connect with, I was still struggling a bit, and I knew that a group's structured
format would be beneficial for further accountability and connections that would also
help me avoid isolating myself.

Still, I didn't really want to make the effort to organize a group. My willpower was flat
in regard to adding anything else to my life. I was already stretched by the normal
activities and rhythm of life. But God continued to nudge me.

Within a couple of weeks, I surrendered to Him. I created a post inviting women to
join a private "accountability group" for "eating with boundaries." Accountability was
the key word. My invitation included that meeting day and time: every Thursday at
5:45 a.m. I thought, *Who would want to show up at 5:45 a.m.?* Truthfully, I chose that
hour because I'd have no excuse for not showing up. Had I chosen mid-morning,
afternoon, or evening, I'd have a pack of excuses to lean on. I was a busy mom with a
full homeschooling schedule and activities—my children's sporting games and events,

homeschool functions, field trips, serving in ministry, working in my husband's business, and other appointments and meetings. There were a lot of moving parts in our family of seven.

The only thing I had going on at 5:45 a.m. was sleeping. Blessed sleep in which I wanted no interference. So yes, I was still hesitant, but I knew I was obeying God's prompting. I needed such a group—and maybe some other women did too.

We formed our group and met every week for almost 5 years. Although we no longer meet at that weekly time due to some scheduling changes, we still communicate throughout the week, sharing our struggles and asking for prayer. We talk about our commitments, individual food plans, and struggles. We each needed help with all three. We became way more than accountability buddies; we became great friends!

Because the group has been such a lifesaver and life-giver for us, I'm sharing with you the accountability group guidelines to make it easier for you to consider creating your group.

Group of Four; One Hour Weekly Meeting

1. Two minutes of greeting and a brief opening prayer acknowledging God's presence and His favor over the group.

2. The first round of sharing is also brief—only about one minute each. Either a member will volunteer to begin, the facilitator will open the round, or members will take turns opening the brief sharing time each week, which sounds like this:

    > I'm feeling . . .
    > My victory this past week was . . .
    > Regarding my commitment from last week, . . .

3. The group then moves into a second, longer round of sharing in the same order, about ten to twelve minutes each, in more detail. We share what's going on in our individual circumstances and ask for advice if desired.

4. Next, the group spends one to three minutes extending feedback with love and encouragement, bearing in mind Hebrews 3:13: "Encourage one another daily, as long as it is called 'Today.'" Every day is today!

5. The final round of sharing is just one minute each and sounds like this:

    > My takeaway is . . .
    > My commitment this week is . . .

6. A group member or the facilitator closes with prayer or a Bible verse for the week.

Yes, a new group's initial meeting can feel awkward, but we know that we'll grow comfortable with each other and feel safe and loved as friendships deepen. Such an accountability group becomes a beautiful place of refuge and encouraging sisterhood of honest accountability regarding our individual decisions and actions (or inactions).

In addition to having a designated or rotating facilitator, one member should volunteer to serve as secretary for at least a set term (like three months, six months, or a year) to fulfill these needs:

- Design and provide the group with a list of meeting dates (covering a span of time like one year or six months) so members are on the same page regarding holidays, etc.
- Track the dates and alert members of any changes.
- Takes brief notes during each meeting, tracking shared commitments, prayer requests, etc.

Know that the enemy will invite himself to every meeting. So remember the armor of God and God's power within you, and pray over your meetings and members in advance. With that in mind, ask the group from the first meeting to commit to the following courtesies in defense against the enemy's nonstop efforts. These courtesies are safeguards against him gaining any entrance to your meetings:

- Be prepared with what you'll share, and watch the time. (Alternatively, the facilitator can also use a timer).
- Silence your phone, put it away, and when others are sharing, mute your mic. Background noises like barking dogs, phone pings and rings, and delivery trucks are very distracting and disruptive.
- Respect and encourage each other.

Prayerfully consider starting and committing to a private online accountability group.

Include the following in your posted announcement:

- facilitator name
- first meeting date
- meeting day of the week
- beginning and ending times

Congratulations!

Great job completing this knowledge-gaining book, a journey of surrendering to God's best for you.

Now what? Continue to stand firm and stay yoked with Christ!

Stay in God's Word—reading, studying, and memorizing.

Stay in prayer and praise to Your heavenly Father.

Stay in the posture of full surrender to God's will, using the tools of surrender.

Stay in the boundaries designed for your utmost health in every regard.

Stay in the armor of God every day, always.

Stay in the posture of receiving and extending God's grace and love.

Stay surrounded by like-minded support sisters.

Stay engaged in sound resources.

Stay connected with Life Unbinged.

Life Unbinged offers several ways to gain tips, truth, recipes, encouragement, support, and much more.

- Visit our website and **sign up to receive by email** our updates and encouragement.
- On our homepage, click our social media links and follow us!
  - YouTube
  - Facebook
  - Instagram

www.lifeunbinged.com

Want deeper support? Join Surrender Sisters.

Surrender Sisters is our private group where you'll experience ongoing connections with women who are living life unbinged. As with any addiction, *staying free* is a continual, intentional, daily walk that reaches far beyond finishing a book, a workbook, or a course. We must continue to use the tools and also stay engaged in ongoing, connective support, encouragement, and accountability with others committed to living life unbinged.

Surrender Sisters is a growing group of women committed to godliness.

- We love the Lord!
- We've become free from the cycles of food obsession.
- We stay deeply rooted in God's Word.
- We're committed to remaining free by keeping God and His Word in the highest place of our hearts and lives, fleeing from temptation, and maintaining food boundaries.
- We're dedicated to supporting each other through our ongoing journey of a life unbinged.

Surrender Sisters offers the following and more:

- biblical coaching and support
- daily posts of encouragement and motivation
- Zoom gatherings on various topics for accountability
- full access to my personal ongoing journey of food failures and successes
- Monday celebration
- Wednesday writing prompt
- Saturday devotional
- Surrender Sisters games (just friendly competitions)
- Surrender Sisters 25 percent discount at all times on every item in our Life Unbinged store

Support — Encouragement — Coaching — Accountability

Let's continue this journey together, moving forward and upward with Christ and each other in godliness. You're going to love the connection, camaraderie, and continuing sisterhood of support—a life of freedom and continually breaking free from the vicious cycle of food addiction.

Learn more here:

Surrender Sisters membership page:
https://lifeunbinged.com/surrender-sisters/

Learn more about Surrender Sisters

Do not be discouraged or grow weary. Keep your face and thoughts turned to Christ, your mind renewed, and keep steadily working on your goals, for your labor in the Lord is not in vain.

(2 Corinthians 4:8–9; 2 Thessalonians 3:13; 1 Corinthians 15:58)

Recommended Resources

The 3-meal plan is ideal and recommended, but the following plans are optional for those who medically need to eat smaller meals more often or prefer longer periods of fasting.

2-Meal Plan:	
Meal 1	**Meal 2**
1 ½ Protein 1 Breakfast Grain 10 oz. Vegetables 1 Fat 1 Fruit	1 ½ Protein 10 oz. Vegetables 1 Fat 1 Fruit

4-Meal Plan:			
Breakfast	**Lunch**	**Mid-Afternoon**	**Dinner**
1 Protein 1 Breakfast Grain 1 Fruit	½ Protein 10 oz. Vegetables 1 Fat	½ Protein 1 Fruit	1 Protein 10 oz. Vegetables or Salad 1 Fat

5-Meal Plan:				
Breakfast	**Mid-Morning**	**Lunch**	**Mid-Afternoon**	**Dinner**
½ Protein ½ Grain ½ Fruit	½ Protein ½ Grain ½ Fruit	Protein 5 oz. Vegetables ½ Fruit ½ Fat	½ Protein 5 oz. Vegetables ½ Fruit ½ Fat	1 Protein 10 oz. Vegetables or Salad 1 Fat

Recommended Resources

Practical Tool

OXO Good Grips 11-pound scale with pull-out display
www.oxo.com/11-lb-stainless-steel-scale-w-pull-out-display.html

Podcast

Taste for Truth podcast, Barb Raveling

App

I Deserve a Donut

Book

Life Unbinged: 2 Week Meal Plan with Recipes and Grocery List
https://lifeunbinged.com/store/

Online Course

Life Unbinged: 60 Day Journey to Surrender
https://lifeunbinged.com/60-day-surrender-course/

Shopping

Tools for Success
https://lifeunbinged.com/store/

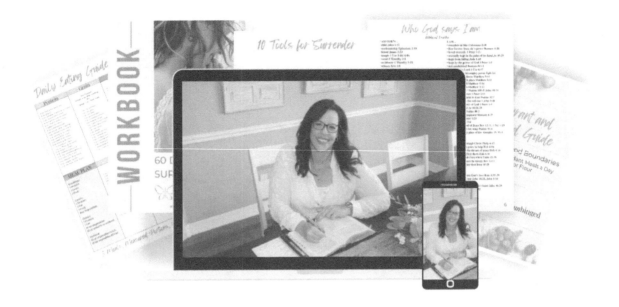

60 DAY JOURNEY TO SURRENDER

Come join the Life Unbinged signature course, Journey to Surrender! With this 60 day course, you can meet weekly with a small group of women who are ready to surrender their food to God. Each small group is led by a Life Unbinged coach, who is there to offer support, guidance, and wisdom as you work through the course material together.

With the online course, you get video teachings covering the topics presented in this book, live monthly coaching with me, as well as a number of fantastic resources that will help you as you commit to a sugar-free, flour-free life.

The small groups offer you the opportunity to talk through, share, and learn from others who are also on the path to freedom from food addiction.

We have groups starting every few months, and we'd love to see you there! Find out more at www.lifeunbinged.com/60-day-surrender-course/.

Notes

1   Chris Carberg, "Food Addiction," AddictionHelp.com, last updated May 10, 2024, https://www.addictionhelp.com/food-addiction/.

2   Nicole M. Avena, Pedro Rada, and Bartley G. Hoebel, abstract for "Evidence for Sugar Addiction: Behavioral and Neurochemical Effects of Intermittent, Excessive Sugar Intake," *Neuroscience and Biobehavioral Reviews* 32, no. 1 (2008): 20. https://www.ncbi.nlm.nih.gov/pmc/articles/PMC2235907/.

3   Qing Yang, "Gain Weight by 'Going Diet?' Artificial Sweeteners and the Neurobiology of Sugar Cravings: Neuroscience 2010," *Yale Journal of Biology and Medicine* 83, no. 2 (June 2010). https://www.ncbi.nlm.nih.gov/pmc/articles/PMC2892765/#!po=59.3750.

4   Chuck Swindoll, "Holding on Loosely," Insight for Living, April 11, 2013, https://insight.org/resources/article-library/individual/holding-on-loosely.

5   *Merriam-Webster*, s.v. "self-serving (*adj.*)," accessed June 28, 2024, https://www.merriam-webster.com/dictionary/self-serving.

6   Jon Smith, "Six Ways Iron Sharpens Iron," Collegiate Disciple Maker, March 25, 2022, https://collegiatedisciplemaker.com/six-ways-iron-sharpens-iron/.

7   *Merriam-Webster*, s.v. "thankful (*adj.*)," accessed June 28, 2024, https://www.merriam-webster.com/dictionary/thankful.

8   *Merriam-Webster*, s.v. "grateful (*adj.*)," accessed June 28, 2024, https://www.merriam-webster.com/dictionary/grateful.

9   Jessie Keith, "10 Worst Garden Weeds and Their Management," Fafard, accessed April 14, 2024, https://fafard.com/managing-the-worst-perennial-weeds/#.

10   Billy Graham, "The Holy Spirit," Billy Graham Evangelistic Association, September 27, 2021, https://billygraham.org/devotion/the-holy-spirit/.

11   *Merriam-Webster*, s.v. "debauchery (*n.*)," accessed June 28, 2024, https://www.merriam-webster.com/dictionary/debauchery.

12   *Merriam-Webster*, s.v. "intention (*n.*)," accessed June 28, 2024, https://www.merriam-webster.com/dictionary/intention.

13   Lana Burgess, "8 Benefits of Crying: Why Do We Cry, and When to Seek Support," Medical News Today, last updated July 13, 2023, https://www.medicalnewstoday.com/articles/319631#benefits-of-crying.

14   Burgess, "8 Benefits of Crying."

15   *Merriam-Webster*, s.v. "grace (*n.*)," accessed June 28, 2024, https://www.merriam-webster.com/dictionary/grace.

16   Scott Hubbard, "Every Sin Hides a Lie: Three Ways Temptation Betrays Us," desiringGod, June 4, 2020, https://www.desiringgod.org/articles/every-sin-hides-a-lie.

17   Hubbard, "Every Sin Hides a Lie."

Made in United States
Cleveland, OH
23 April 2025

16293916R00122